Preservation Rhinoplasty Merges with Structure Rhinoplasty

Editor

DEAN M. TORIUMI

FACIAL PLASTIC SURGERY CLINICS OF NORTH AMERICA

www.facialplastic.theclinics.com

Consulting Editor
ANTHONY P. SCLAFANI

February 2023 • Volume 31 • Number 1

ELSEVIER

1600 John F. Kennedy Boulevard • Suite 1800 • Philadelphia, Pennsylvania, 19103-2899

http://www.theclinics.com

**FACIAL PLASTIC SURGERY CLINICS OF NORTH AMERICA Volume 31, Number 1
February 2023 ISSN 1064-7406, ISBN-13: 978-0-323-94017-7**

Editor: Stacy Eastman
Developmental Editor: Ann Gielou M. Posedio

Facial Plastic Surgery Clinics of North America (ISSN 1064-7406) is published quarterly by Elsevier Inc., 360 Park Avenue South, New York, NY 10010-1710. Months of issue are February, May, August, and November. Business and Editorial Offices: 1600 John F. Kennedy Blvd., Suite 1800, Philadelphia, PA 19103-2899. Periodicals postage paid at New York, NY, and additional mailing offices. Subscription prices are $428.00 per year (US individuals), $728.00 per year (US institutions), $477.00 per year (Canadian individuals), $904.00 per year (Canadian institutions), $568.00 per year (foreign individuals), $904.00 per year (foreign institutions), $100.00 per year (US students), $100.00 per year (Canadian students), and $255.00 per year (foreign students). Foreign air speed delivery is included in all *Clinics* subscription prices. All prices are subject to change without notice. POSTMASTER: Send address changes to *Facial Plastic Surgery Clinics*, Elsevier Health Sciences Division, Subscription Customer Service, 3251 Riverport Lane, Maryland Heights, MO 63043. **Customer service: 1-800-654-2452 (US and Canada); 1-314-447-8871 (outside US and Canada); Fax: 314-447-8029; E-mail: journalscustomerservice-usa@elsevier.com (for print support); journalsonlinesupport-usa@elsevier.com (for online support).**

Reprints. For copies of 100 or more of articles in this publication, please contact the Commercial Reprints Department, Elsevier Inc., 360 Park Avenue South, New York, NY 10010-1710. Tel.: 212-633-3874; Fax: 212-633-3820; E-mail: reprints@elsevier.com.

Facial Plastic Surgery Clinics of North America is covered in *MEDLINE/PubMed* (*Index Medicus*).

Contributors

CONSULTING EDITOR

ANTHONY P. SCLAFANI, MD, MBA, FACS
Professor, Department of Otolaryngology–
Head and Neck Surgery, Weill Cornell
Medicine, Director of Facial Plastic Surgery,
NewYork-Presbyterian/Weill Cornell Medical
Center, New York, New York, USA

EDITOR

DEAN M. TORIUMI, MD
Professor, Department of Otolaryngology–
Head and Neck Surgery, Rush University
Medical School, Private Practice, Toriumi
Facial Plastics, Chicago, Illinois, USA

AUTHORS

DIEGO ARANCIBIA-TAGLE, MD
International and European Board Certified in
Facial Plastic and Reconstructive Surgery
(IBCFPRS - EBCFPRS), Fellow of The
European Board of Otorhinolaryngology–Head
and Neck Surgery (FEBORL).
Otorhinolaryngology–Head and Neck Surgery
Specialist, Private Practice, Mallorca,
Spain

BARIŞ ÇAKIR
Associate Professor, Teswvikiye Cd., Siswli,
Istanbul, Turkey

WILSON J. DEWES, MD
Department of Facial Plastic Surgery, FUNDEF
and Clinica Wilson Dewes, Lajeado, Brazil

OZAN EROL, MD
Fellow of The European Academy of Facial
Plastic Surgery, Fellow of The European Board
of Otorhinolaryngology–Head and Neck
Surgery (FEBORL), Otorhinolaryngology–Head
and Neck Surgery Specialist, Istanbul,
Turkey

MARIO BAZANELLI JUNQUEIRA FERRAZ, MD
Department of Facial Plastic Surgery, Clinica
Mario Ferraz, Campinas, Brazil

MIGUEL GONÇALVES FERREIRA, MD, PhD
Centro Hospitalar Universitário do Porto,
Instituto de Ciências Biomédicas Abel Salazar -
Universidade do Porto, Hospital da Luz -
Arrábida, Clínica do Nariz e Face, Porto,
Portugal

VALERIO FINOCCHI, MD
Private Practitioner, MySelf Clinic, Roma, Italy

BÜLENT GENÇ, MD
Private Practice, Caddebostan Mah Çam
Fıstığı Sok, Istanbul, Turkey

OLIVIER GERBAULT, MD
Chairman, Plastic Surgery, PEMV, Vincennes -
Paris, France, Visiting Professor of the ISAPS,
Vice president of the Rhinoplasty Society of
Europe

ABDULKADIR GOKSEL, MD
RinoIstanbul Facial Plastic Surgery Clinic,
Istanbul, Turkey

SEBASTIAN HAACK, MD
Private Practice, Böheimstraße, Stuttgart,
Germany

EMRE ILHAN, MD
International and European Board Certified in
Facial Plastic and Reconstructive Surgery
(IBCFPRS - EBCFPRS), Otorhinolaryngology–
Head and Neck Surgery Specialist, Private
Practice, Istanbul, Turkey

LUIZ CARLOS ISHIDA, MD, PhD
Plastic Surgery Division, University of São
Paulo, São Paulo, Brazil

MILOS KOVACEVIC, MD
Private Practice, Hamburg, Germany

SAM P. MOST, MD
Division of Facial Plastic and Reconstructive
Surgery, Stanford University School of
Medicine, Stanford, California, USA

JOSE CARLOS NEVES, MD
International and European Board Certified in
Facial Plastic and Reconstructive Surgery
(IBCFPRS - EBCFPRS), Otorhinolaryngology–
Head and Neck Surgery Specialist, Private
Practice at MYFACE Clinic and Academy,
Lisbon, Portugal

PRIYESH N. PATEL, MD
Division of Facial Plastic and Reconstructive
Surgery, Department of Otolaryngology,
Vanderbilt University Medical Center,
Nashville, Tennessee, USA

YVES SABAN, MD
Private Practice, Nice, France, USA

MASOUD SAMAN, MD
Saman Facial Plastic Surgery, PLLC,
New York, New York, USA

MARILINE SANTOS, MD
Centro Hospitalar Universitário do
Porto, Instituto de Ciências Biomédicas
Abel Salazar - Universidade do Porto, Porto,
Portugal

**GUILHERME CONSTANTE
PREIS SELLA, MD, PhD**
Department of Facial Plastic Surgery, Clinica
Sella, Maringa, Brazil

J. REGAN THOMAS, MD
Emeritus Professor, Facial Plastic and
Reconstructive Surgery, Northwestern
University School of Medicine, Chicago,
Illinois; Visiting Professor, Facial Plastic and
Reconstructive Surgery, University of New
Mexico School of Medicine, Albuquerque,
New Mexico

DEAN M. TORIUMI, MD
Professor, Department of Otolaryngology–
Head and Neck Surgery, Rush University
Medical School, Private Practice, Toriumi
Facial Plastics, Chicago, Illinois,
USA

KHANH NGOC TRAN, MBBS
RinoIstanbul Facial Plastic Surgery Clinic,
Istanbul, Turkey

VALENTINO VELLONE, MD, PhD
Department of Maxillofacial Surgery, "S.
Maria" Hospital, Terni, Italy

Contents

Overview of Dorsal Preservation Rhinoplasty 1

Priyesh N. Patel and Sam P. Most

> Renewed interest in dorsal preservation rhinoplasty (DPR) stems from theoretic esthetic and functional advantages over conventional hump resection. DPR fundamentally consists of en bloc dorsal lowering via a combined septal resection and mobilization of the bony pyramid. Several technical modifications exist, allowing for the expansion of DPR indications. Although studies suggest success with these techniques, comparative data to conventional hump resection are limited. Challenges and stigmata of DPR include a radix step-off, hump recurrence, supratip saddling, and widening of the midvault. The fusion of structural techniques with preservation ideology will facilitate the incorporation of DPR into clinical practice.

Long-Term Follow-Up with Dorsal Preservation Rhinoplasty 13

Masoud Saman and Yves Saban

> The rapid resurgence of interest in performance of dorsal preservation (DP) rhinoplasty techniques in recent years has come with scarcity of data for long-term outcomes. In this article, the authors aim to contribute to preservation rhinoplasty (PR) literature by providing long-term follow-up with dorsal preservation, specifically presenting data related to superior strip DP functional and esthetic complications, followed by a detailed analysis of the same.

My Approach to Preservation Rhinoplasty 25

Barış Çakır, Bülent Genç, Valerio Finocchi, and Sebastian Haack

> Preservation rhinoplasty entails the preservation of the supportive ligaments, preservation of the cartilage structure, and preserving the anatomy of the nasal dorsum. The preservation methods I use are described in this article.

Surface Techniques in Dorsal Preservation 45

Miguel Gonçalves Ferreira and Mariline Santos

> Classical dorsal preservation rhinoplasty is typically done with impaction osteotomies (push/let down) and a low septal strip. These approaches are potentially highly

destabilizing maneuvers in the architecture of the nasal pyramid. This is one of the reasons why these approaches did not have a popular acceptance in the 1960s and 1970s. More recently, the surgeon interested in preservation rhinoplasty has the possibility to do so with surface techniques with more control and, if needed, is easily converted to the standard structured techniques if the surgeon does not feel safe with the procedure.

Preservation rhinoplasty represents a growing shift in rhinoplasty philosophy toward preserving structurally sound anatomy and reshaping existing nasal structures into esthetic and functional ideals. The preservation technique is made more accessible by the open approach, which provides an opportunity for the deformity to be clearly visualized from the tip of the nose to the dorsum, as well as enables greater ease of powered instrument access. The addition of the Piezo-electric device, with its range of rhinoplasty inserts, enables more precise and accurate management of the osseocartilaginous vault, reduces the risk of surface irregularities, and hence optimizes the overall surgical outcome.

 Video content accompanies this article at http://www.facialplastic.theclinics.com.

Dorsal preservation involves eliminating the dorsal hump by performing reduction while preserving the patient's natural dorsal anatomy. This can involve surface manipulation or foundational techniques or a combination of both. When surgeons begin performing dorsal preservation, there are important factors to consider to avoid complications. In an effort to inform surgeons on how to avoid unfavorable outcomes, I will discuss my first 20 cases where I performed dorsal preservation. I review less than ideal outcomes and how these issues can be prevented.

 Video content accompanies this article at http://www.facialplastic.theclinics.com.

Severe septal deviations are a constant challenge for rhinosurgeons. As the septum is the most important pillar of the nasal framework, septal deformities require correction to insure a straight nose. The septum should be on the midline without any tension to ensure a correct healing of the external nasal pyramid. In certain cases, the association of a correct septoplasty and dorsal preservation allows the treatment of the crooked nose and at the same time gives natural results with rapid postoperative recovery. The aim of this article was to underline the versatility of the dorsal preservation technique for the correction of severe septal deviation.

 Video content accompanies this article at http://www.facialplastic.theclinics.com.

The subdorsal cantilever graft (SDCG) is a costal cartilage graft that is positioned below the nasal dorsum to control the position of the nasal bones and middle nasal vault. SDCG type A is used to raise the middle nasal vault and caudal nasal bones to correct the saddle nose deformity. SDCG type B can be used to raise the entire dorsum of the nose (radix, bony vault, and middle vault) in the ethnic augmentation rhinoplasty patient. This article will discuss the indications and technique of the SDCG in dorsal preservation rhinoplasty.

Brazilian Approach to Dorsum Preservation

Mario Bazanelli Junqueira Ferraz, Wilson J. Dewes, Luiz Carlos Ishida, and Guilherme Constante Preis Sella

Brazil has always been a fertile place for plastic surgery techniques, especially cosmetic, and it was not different in rhinoplasty. In Brazil surgeons started using the dorsal preservation rhinoplasty in the 1970s. Techniques have changed, the problems and contraindications were challenged, and solutions proposed. As a result, indications were expanded to almost every kind of nose. Surface working executed with power tools, such as the piezoelectric device and the power drill, complemented the techniques and allowed for refinement in execution. Today the Brazilian preservation techniques are adopted and improved by many surgeons around the world.

Ultrasonic Rhinoplasty and Septoplasty for Dorsum Preservation and for Dorsum Structural Reconstruction

Olivier Gerbault

Ultrasonic rhinoplasty and ultrasonic septoplasty reshape the nasal bones using piezoelectric instruments specifically developed for these operations. They allow the realization of precise osteotomies under direct visual control after having performed first an open or closed extended approach, but also ostectomies and rhinosculpture. Piezoelectric instruments preserve bone stability by not damaging bone support structures and avoiding unwanted fractures. They allow precise control of nasal bone movements, their orientation, and their final position. The different inserts of ultrasonic rhinoplasty and ultrasonic septoplasty are detailed, with their scope of action. The applications to dorsum preservation and structural remodeling of dorsum are presented.

Precision Segmental Preservation Rhinoplasty: Avoiding Widening, Defining New Dorsal Esthetic Lines in Dorsal Preservation Rhinoplasty

Jose Carlos Neves, Ozan Erol, Diego Arancibia-Tagle, and Emre Ilhan

 Video content accompanies this article at http://www.facialplastic.theclinics.com.

Experiencing great worldwide scientific excitement, the number of nose preservation surgeries has increased rapidly, promoting a considerable percentage of drawbacks and complications, causing many surgeons to recoil and return to classic resective techniques. In this study, we develop concepts that allow us to operate noses with preservation rhinoplasty that were previously considered to be among the absolute contraindications. Redefining new dorsal aesthetic lines, controlling the nasal lateral wall and the naso-facial groove surfaces, avoiding mid-vault widening and being precise in the design of bony and cartilaginous nasal profile, avoiding any type of irregularity, are strategies that will be presented.

FACIAL PLASTIC SURGERY CLINICS OF NORTH AMERICA

SERIES OF RELATED INTEREST

Clinics in Plastic Surgery
https://www.plasticsurgery.theclinics.com
Otolaryngologic Clinics
https://www.oto.theclinics.com
Dermatologic Clinics
https://www.derm.theclinics.com

THE CLINICS ARE AVAILABLE ONLINE!
Access your subscription at:
www.theclinics.com

Farewell

CONSULTING EDITOR FAREWELL

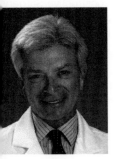

J. Regan Thomas, MD
Editor

It is fortunately surprising, and perhaps difficult to believe presently, that there was a period in the history of our specialty of facial plastic and reconstructive surgery where we were not recognized or represented as a specialty through a journal or identified publication. Indeed, Facial Plastic Surgery as a specific entity was being actively opposed by several other identifiable specialty groups and even by some individuals within Otolaryngology. Individual physicians who wished to focus on facial plastic and reconstructive surgery procedures and were inspired to further expand and develop expertise in that direction at that time had very few outlets and opportunities to share experience or interact with others of complementary and comparable interest.

With those issues in mind, an insightful discussion during a social dinner occasion led Dr Wayne Larrabee and me to consider that a key step in strengthening and gaining further recognition for facial plastic surgery would be to develop a specialty-specific medical journal. With that conclusion in mind, a publisher was contacted and discussions were provided, which led to the agreement to publish on a regular basis the identifiable, specialty-specific and recognized medical journal, *Facial Plastic Surgery Clinics of North America*. The first dedicated facial plastic surgery journal was published.

Dr Larrabee and I were initially coeditors, and we established an editorial review board. Full-time publisher staff members were identified and assigned to the *Facial Plastic Surgery Clinics of North America* team, and the journal soon became a recognizable and academically appreciated entity. Dr Larrabee and I also worked with others through the AMA process to establish a second facial plastic journal, which after numerous political steps successfully evolved, and Dr Larrabee left the *Facial Plastic Surgery Clinics of North America* to be editor of the then AMA *Archives* journal.

As the physician editor of *Facial Plastic Surgery Clinics of North America* for over 30 years, I am genuinely proud to see the journal's impact and recognition be identified internationally. The clinical articles of the journal's many expert contributing authors have become a useful resource for specialty education and training. Likewise, it is a frequent and valuable resource for maintenance of individual skills as well as comparative evaluation of the activities of our colleagues and specialty overall.

On a personal note, I have reached a point in a successful and very enjoyable career where some aspects of professional retirement seem appropriate. I am stepping down as Consulting Editor for *Facial Plastic Surgery Clinics of North America*. I am very proud of the growth and impact the *Facial Plastic Surgery Clinics of North America* have had over the past 30 years. I am genuinely appreciative of the great many publishable contributions of our

Facial Plast Surg Clin N Am 31 (2023) ix–x
https://doi.org/10.1016/j.fsc.2022.09.003
1064-7406/23/© 2022 Published by Elsevier Inc.

many guest editors and contributing authors. Certainly, I absolutely appreciate the expertise and commitment of the members of the Elsevier team, who are always there to see to the continuing success of the *Facial Plastic Surgery Clinics of North America*.

I am indeed very proud and pleased to have had a role in the establishment, growth, and ongoing presence of the *Facial Plastic Surgery Clinics of North America*. I look forward to its ongoing impact on the expertise and recognition of the surgical specialty of Facial Plastic and Reconstructive Surgery.

J. Regan Thomas, MD
Facial Plastic and Reconstructive Surgery
Northwestern University School of Medicine
60 East Delaware Place
Chicago, IL 60611
USA

E-mail address:
regan.thomas@nm.org

Tribute
Hail and Farewell!

After 30 years, J. Regan Thomas, MD steps down as Editor of *Facial Plastic Surgery Clinics of North America*. Dr Thomas has been the Editor of the *Facial Plastic Surgery Clinics of North America* since its inception in 1993. We thank Dr Thomas not only for his efforts in leading *Facial Plastic Surgery Clinics of North America* but also as someone who helped create a strong scientific, academic, and clinical foundation for Facial Plastic Surgery. As a clinician, teacher, researcher, administrator, and always an advocate, Dr Thomas has been instrumental in cementing the position of Facial Plastic and Reconstructive Surgery in the medical and lay communities in North America and around the world. More senior readers will remember a time when otolaryngology training programs had no faculty dedicated to Facial Plastic Surgery; when Facial Plastic Surgery had little to no voice in organized medicine; when a facial plastic surgeon was disparaged as "just an ENT" by other specialties and the public; when hospitals were reticent to credential facial plastic surgeons in the very procedures we, as a specialty, pioneered and refined. Dr Thomas' calm, insightful, and endearingly persistent approach helped define and establish Facial Plastic and Reconstructive Surgery as an essential part of Medicine (**Fig. 1**).

Born in Joplin, Missouri, Dr Thomas graduated from Drury College, where he was Student Body President, and the University of Missouri School of Medicine (MU). He did his surgical residency at Yale University and his otolaryngology residency at MU. Two events during his early years had a major impact on his life and career. At Drury, he met Rhonda Churchill, and they were married following graduation in 1969. Early in his medical career, he met Gene Tardy and completed a fellowship in Facial Plastic Surgery with Gene at Northwestern University in 1979. That fellowship provided a springboard for his passion for Facial Plastic Surgery and his own commitment to training talented young physicians through his fellowship programs for the next 43 years.

M. Eugene Tardy Jr MD: "As the very first of my valued fellows, Dr. Thomas has established himself as one of the most creative, effective and talented facial plastic surgeons of our time. Creative surgeon, mesmerizing teacher and a warm physician's touch characterize his attributes: his devotion to the Aequanimitas tradition of medical excellence sets the standard for others. To his

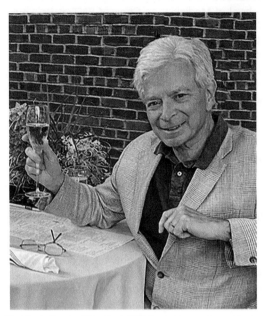

Fig. 1. J. Regan Thomas, MD.

credit, Regan has never known a stranger, generously sharing his knowledge, expertise and friendship to all with whom he is associated. His leadership in the development of Facial Plastic Surgery world-wide is exemplary" (**Fig. 2**).

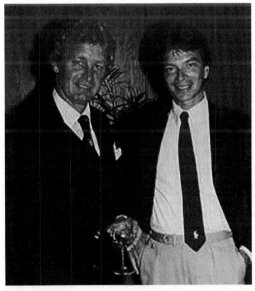

Fig. 2. Drs M. Eugene Tardy Jr (*left*) and J. Regan Thomas (*right*).

Facial Plast Surg Clin N Am 31 (2023) xi–xiv
https://doi.org/10.1016/j.fsc.2022.09.005
1064-7406/23/© 2022 Published by Elsevier Inc.

Dr Thomas has served on the faculty of six major academic otolaryngology departments, including MU, and served as Director of Facial Plastic and Reconstructive Surgery at Washington University School of Medicine, as Chair of ENT at St. Louis University for 6 years and at the University of Illinois–Chicago (UIC) for 18 years, as professor at Northwestern University School of Medicine, where he was appointed Professor Emeritus on his retirement this summer, and as Visiting Professor at New Mexico University School of Medicine.

A man of many talents, Dr Thomas was a multitasker before it became popular. Running a successful cosmetic and reconstructive surgery practice while writing, editing, and publishing extensively and even serving as an on-air TV medical reporter on ABC and NBC would be more than a full-time job for most; beyond these responsibilities, Dr Thomas was a full-time teacher. Thirty-five American Academy of Facial Plastic & Reconstructive Surgery (AAFPRS) fellows have trained with Dr Thomas, and many have continued in Regan's footsteps by serving as fellowship directors. His fellows have continued his tradition of calm, compassionate patient care, service, and teaching, whether in private practice, academic medicine, or medical administration, and they are a source of great pride to Regan.

In addition, Dr Thomas has lectured and trained physicians across the United States and around the world. He has made more than 300 scholarly presentations, serving as an international ambassador for the Academy and specialty with casual charm and understated brilliance.

Regan has written over 270 publications, authored seven textbooks, and in addition to his work on *Facial Plastic Surgery Clinics of North America*, has served on the editorial boards of *Archives of Facial Plastic Surgery*, *Laryngoscope*, and *Otolaryngology–Head & Neck Surgery*, helping to build an independent presence for Facial Plastic Surgery while remaining collaborative within otolaryngology.

Dr Thomas' publications and presentations often include tributes to his family: his partner in life, Rhonda, and their three children and their families. As Regan has written, "*My wife, Rhonda Churchill Thomas, deserves my ongoing appreciation and gratitude for her enthusiastic and always present support for my professional activities. Likewise, I offer my sincere appreciation to my children, Ryan, Aaron, and Evan, for their inspiration and example*" (**Figs. 3–6**).

Dr Thomas has served the local, national, and international communities as President of the AAFPRS, the American Academy of Otolaryngology–Head and Neck Surgery (AAO-

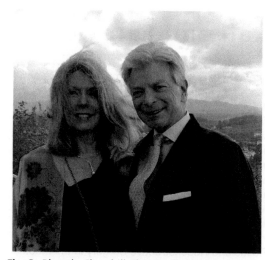

Fig. 3. Rhonda Churchill Thomas (*left*) with J. Regan Thomas (*right*).

HNS), the American Board of Facial Plastic & Reconstructive Surgery, the Illinois State Medical Society, and as Chair of the Illinois Medical Society and National ENT PACs. His awards are too numerous to list but include Alumni awards from Drury College and MU, Honor awards from the AAFPRS, AAO-HNS, and the Mexican Society of Rhinology and Facial Plastic Surgery, Mentor of the Year award from the AAO-HNS, and the Jacques Joseph award from the European Academy of Facial Plastic Surgery. He was named Teacher of the Year by his residents at both UIC and Northwestern.

Dr Thomas has served patients for 50 years, developing safe procedures and medical techniques in Facial Plastic Surgery (the "safety face lift"), reconstructive surgery repairing trauma and cancer defects, and scar revision. He is touched

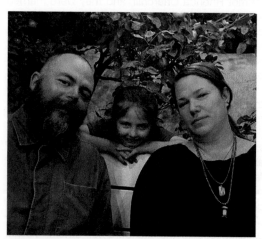

Fig. 4. Dr Thomas' son Aaron (*left*) with granddaughter Levi (*center*) and Lisa.

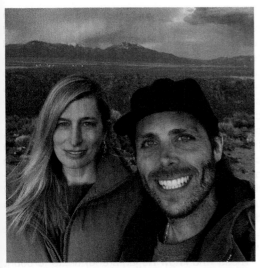

Fig. 5. Dr Thomas' daughter, Ryan (*left*), with Martim.

to treat multiple generations and relatives of patients from the same family.

What makes Dr Thomas a role model is his devotion to advancing the field and to building the Facial Plastic Surgery community, locally and internationally. His early advocacy on behalf of the AAFPRS helped establish our field's position in organized medicine. Working with other giants of the field, Dr Thomas has been a strong advocate for us by strength of argument as well as by his ability to reach across aisles, fields, and borders to establish a robust and interconnected Facial Plastic Surgery community.

Many of his fellows, trainees, and peers have offered their appreciation and praise for Dr Thomas. In this limited space, we are only able to include a few thoughts from some of those from around the world who know him well.

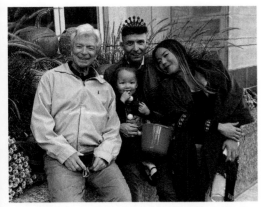

Fig. 6. Dr Thomas (*left*) with son Evan, granddaughter Aika, and Leah.

Steve Perkins, MD (US): "I consider Regan Thomas as one of my closest and career-long best friends and a colleague with extremely mutual views on the field of Facial Plastic Surgery. While traveling the States and the world together teaching Facial Plastic Surgery, we became extremely close friends with mutual interests in skiing, racing cars, boating, and golf. Always we have enjoyed dinners together with our international friends and partaking in the joys of all kinds of wine!"

Gilbert Nolste Trenite, MD (Amsterdam): "Regan's legacy of Facial Plastic Surgery, through his books, articles and training of fellows who had the privilege to learn from him, will stay. Many colleagues over the world will miss his excellent lectures. Regan is a born teacher. I am proud to be his friend and "brother" as he calls me. We both know that there is more in life than a brilliant career."

Wayne Larrabee, MD (US): "Regan possessed the breadth of knowledge and diplomatic skills we needed to make The Clinics successful and it has continued to be successful to this day. It has been an honor and great pleasure to have worked with Regan most of my career. I wish him well in retirement but also know he will continue to contribute in many ways."

Roxana Cobo, MD (Colombia): "Friend, teacher, adviser, role model, thoughtful leader….all of these are words that describe Regan Thomas. His generosity in sharing his knowledge and promoting Facial Plastic Surgery around the world is something I will never forget and will be forever thankful. All the international community will miss Regan, thanks for giving us so much!"

Hesham Saleh, MD (London): "I met Regan many years ago in an international conference, and it struck me how eloquently he delivered lectures on complex subjects, making them easily accessible to all. At the same time, he had immense warmth and an ability to make those of us with much less experience feel good about themselves. For all these years Regan continued to be an outstanding surgeon, amazing teacher, vast researcher and, above all, a wonderful friend."

Jose A Patrocinio, MD (Brazil): "Those angels who enlighten our lives with light of knowledge, curiosity and wisdom are TEACHERS! Regan is an angel!"

Efrain Davalos, MD (Mexico): "Regan Thomas is my second father, my mentor, and my example to follow in Facial Plastic Surgery and in many other aspects in life. One of the most famous facial plastic surgeons worldwide, who is always willing and ready to encourage and teach people from all over the world with his depths of knowledge and enthusiasm. But I just call him 'El Jefe.'"

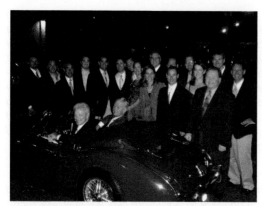

Fig. 7. Dr Thomas and Dr M. Eugene Tardy Jr (*in car*) with Dr Thomas' fellows.

Yong Ju Jang (South Korea): "*Dr. Regan Thomas is a true giant in Facial Plastic Surgery. His lifelong teaching to colleagues and service to patients will leave a huge mark in the history of Facial Plastic Surgery. Personally, I am blessed to have known him as a close friend and professional colleague for over 12 years. He is a real exemplary 'American gentleman' with a great personality and a sense of humor and his legacy will endure.*"

Peter A. Adamson, MD (Canada): "*Regan reflects the character and professionalism that all facial plastic surgeons should aspire to. And he does this with a twinkle in his eye and a wicked sense of humor. I always remember and cherish our verbal repartees. The best of friends, the best of times, the best of memories.*"

Unfortunately, space limits the comments we can include here. Those who have met or listened to Dr Thomas know his keen intellect and careful reasoning, always keeping the patient as his primary concern. As a Thomas fellow (**Fig. 7**), I write here on behalf of those who have worked with and studied under Dr Thomas, who know and appreciate his warmth and kindness, his southwest Missouri aphorisms, his appreciation of music, art, fine wine, Sprite, McDonald's, and chocolate chip cookies. We learned from him the elegance of a meticulously elevated flap, the graceful subtlety of a carefully contoured nose, the many uses of cotton-tipped applicators, and how to discretely slip out of the office and enjoy a St. Louis Cardinals game on a sunny summer weekday.

Those who know Regan are fortunate to count him as a friend. In Regan, we have a second brother/father, confidant, often coconspirator, and occasional therapist, someone we can count on for advice, support, and the ego check we all occasionally need. *Facial Plastic Surgery Clinics of North America* will continue to uphold the high standards and tenets Dr Thomas has set: refining, advancing, and sharing innovations in the art and science of Facial Plastic and Reconstructive Surgery. I write on behalf of all of us to thank Dr Thomas and acknowledge him as a giant, atop whose shoulders we stand to see a little farther beyond the horizon.

Anthony P. Sclafani, MD, MBA, FACS

Foreword
Fads, Progress, and Paradigm Shifts

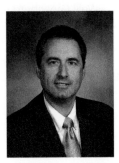

Anthony P. Sclafani, MD, MBA, FACS
Consulting Editor

Strategic Inflection Point: An event that changes the way we think and act.
        —*Andy Grove (co-founder, Intel Corp)*

The Edison Illuminating Company was established in 1882 to provide direct current electricity to power indoor incandescent lights. Nikola Tesla emigrated to the United States in 1884, having already experimented with alternating current and constructed his first induction motor. After briefly working for Thomas Edison, Tesla licensed (and later gave) his patent rights to George Westinghouse. After a bruising commercial and public relations struggle, successfully illuminating the 1893 Chicago World's Fair with alternating current and harnessing the power of Niagara Falls to create electricity, Westinghouse and alternating current had won the "Battle of the Currents."

Along a similar timeline, modern rhinoplasty developed to reduce large noses. John Orlando Roe described correction of the "pug nose" deformity in 1887 and a dorsal reduction in 1891. Weir performed dorsal reduction on a patient in 1892. Jacques Joseph performed his first rhinoplasty in 1898 and published his first text on rhinoplasty in 1912. These surgeons highlighted the technique of dorsal reduction and resection to correct large noses. Concurrently, Goodale performed the first dorsal preservation rhinoplasty in 1898. Others followed, but particularly after the publication of Joseph's textbook, dorsal reduction was ascendant, and dorsal preservation was infrequently performed. While the external approach to rhinoplasty was initiated by Rethi's description of the columellar incision in 1921, endonasal rhinoplasty remained the predominant method approach to rhinoplasty.

History is rarely simple and linear. With the advent of a digital society in the 1970s, direct current has risen to greater importance, as it provides the storable, highly stable, low-voltage current required by personal electronics, such as computers and cellphones, and yes, even electric vehicles. With the work of Padovan and Goodman in the 1970s, external approach rhinoplasty steadily became more common. Subsequent work by Johnson and Toriumi emphasized the importance of structural integrity in rhinoplasty performed through the external approach. The work of Saban and others over the past 15 years in understanding and refining dorsal preservation rhinoplasty has once again brought it to the fore, and patients now frequently present to the office requesting "preservation" surgery. What is old is new again, facilitated by an enhanced understanding of the nose.

It is still quite unclear if we stand at an inflection point in rhinoplasty. I do not seek to give pride of place to one or the other technique. However, a wider, more informed perspective on nasal surgery is of value to any rhinoplasty surgeon. We are at our best when we integrate and synthesize new and old, creating and delivering to our patients the most effective treatments we can tailor to each individual. "Different" need not mean "opposing."

Dr Toriumi has assembled in this issue of *Facial Plastic Surgery Clinics of North America* an

Facial Plast Surg Clin N Am 31 (2023) xv–xvi
https://doi.org/10.1016/j.fsc.2022.09.004

outstanding group of authors who describe their viewpoints and preservation rhinoplasty techniques to provide their patients with outstanding results. These authors provide clear, honest, and frank descriptions of their patient selection and preservation techniques. You may or may not embrace this philosophy and technique, but a better understanding of preservation rhinoplasty will enhance your understanding of the art and science of rhinoplasty. I implore you to keep an open mind, read and enjoy this issue—it is a "must read" for every rhinoplasty surgeon!

Anthony P. Sclafani, MD, MBA, FACS
Department of Otolaryngology
Weill Cornell Medicine
Weill Greenberg Center
1305 York Avenue, Suite Y-5
New York, NY 10021, USA

E-mail address:
ANS9243@MED.CORNELL.EDU

Preface
Preservation Rhinoplasty Merges with Structure Rhinoplasty

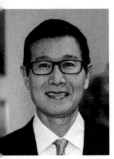

Dean M. Toriumi, MD
Editor

Preservation rhinoplasty is making a resurgence worldwide as surgeons see the benefits of minimizing disruption of key anatomic structures of the nose. The descriptive title, "preservation rhinoplasty," was coined by Rollin K. Daniel,[1] and he and other leaders have initiated a resurgence in recent years. Preservation rhinoplasty encompasses a subperichondrial/subperiosteal dissection plane with preservation of the ligamentous supportive structures, maintenance of the alar cartilages integrity with reshaping performed primarily through tip suturing, and preserving the natural nasal dorsum with possible minor surface modification without creating an "open roof deformity." Dorsal preservation was initially introduced many years ago by Goodale in 1899, Lothrop in 1914, and Cottle in 1946.[2] Wilson Dewes described the Septum Pyramidal Adjustment and Repositioning (SPAR A, B, and C) technique in 2013.[3] Most would agree that Yves Saban led the present resurgence of dorsal preservation.[4] There have been instances where dorsal preservation was promoted in the past with less than enthusiastic fervor. What appears to be different in this movement is that expert surgeons experienced in dorsal preservation are getting outstanding results consistently and are making an effort to teach the techniques worldwide. With the onset of COVID-19 and lockdowns, many of these prominent surgeons were able to spread the message about dorsal preservation through online webinars open to anyone who was interested.

There were multiple lineages where dorsal preservation was taught. These schools taught many surgeons who have become present-day leaders in the preservation movement. Many of these surgeons have contributed to this issue of the *Facial Plastic Surgery Clinics of North America*. I am pleased to have the opportunity to get to know this group of individuals and to learn from those who came from the different lineages (Pinto, Dewes, Ishida, Lopez, Gola, Sulcenti, Saban, Ignacio, Tasca, Carbajal, deLuca, and so forth).

With this present-day resurgence of dorsal preservation, surgeons introduced new innovative techniques to manage the dorsal hump. In this issue, most all the different techniques will be covered. Sam Most provides an overview of dorsal preservation and discusses his approach to the intermediate strip. Yves Saban discusses the high strip and provides his long-term outcomes using this technique. Baris Cakir describes his technique and how he performs endonasal preservation rhinoplasty. Miguel Ferreira discusses the spare roof technique and surface modifications to manage the dorsal hump. Abdulkadir Goksel presents his methods using the open approach and the impact of the "Ballerina maneuver." I discuss my early experience with dorsal preservation, pointing out important nuances to help those who are just starting with this approach. Valerio

Facial Plast Surg Clin N Am 31 (2023) xvii–xviii
https://doi.org/10.1016/j.fsc.2022.08.013

Finocchi covers his SPQR technique and provides specific details on how to execute this technique effectively. Milos Kovacevic and I discuss how the subdorsal cantilever graft can be used in dorsal preservation. Mario Ferraz discusses the Brazilian approach and SPAR and the many lineages of dorsal preservation. Olivier Gerbault provides a clear perspective on piezo technology and how he uses it in his practice.

I am honored to be able to bring this talented group of rhinoplasty surgeons together to teach us all about the nuances of dorsal preservation.

Dean M. Toriumi, MD
Private Practice
60 East Delaware Place, Suite 1425
Chicago, IL 60611, USA

E-mail address:
deantoriumi@toriumimd.com

REFERENCES

1. Daniel RK. The Preservation rhinoplasty: a new rhinoplasty revolution. Aesthet Surg J 2018;38:228–9.
2. Daniel RK, Palhazi P, Saban Y, et al. Preservation rhinoplasty. 3rd edition. Istanbul, Turkey: Septum Publishing; 2020.
3. Ferraz MBJ, Zappelini CEM, Carvalho GM, et al. Cirurgia conservadora do dorso nasal—a filosofia do reposicionamento e ajuste do septo piramidal (SPAR). Rev Bras Cir Cabeça Pescoço 2013;42:124–30.
4. Saban Y, Daniel RK, Polselli R, et al. Dorsal preservation: the push down technique reassessed. Aesthetic Surg J 2018;38:117–31.

Overview of Dorsal Preservation Rhinoplasty

Priyesh N. Patel, MD[a], Sam P. Most, MD[b],*

KEYWORDS

- Dorsal preservation rhinoplasty • Dorsal hump • Structural preservation

KEY POINTS

- The en-bloc treatment of the nasal vault without disruption of the nasal keystone and dorsal esthetic lines has functional and esthetic benefits.
- Dorsal preservation can be combined with open structural methods.
- Although the push-down (PD) and let-down (LD) are two primary techniques used to manage the osseous nasal vault, several modifications exist.
- The variations in septal techniques in dorsal preservation rhinoplasty (DPR) can be categorized by the location of septal cartilage resection and preserved shapes of subdorsal cartilage.
- Several techniques exist to minimize the stigmata of DPR including hump recurrence, mid-vault widening, and radix step-offs.

INTRODUCTION

Global interest in the preservation rhinoplasty has grown significantly following an editorial by Daniel in which relatively destructive rhinoplasty techniques were called into question.[1] Although preservation has been championed by several surgeons across the world for many years, resective and structural methodology has been pervasive.[2] Contemporary preservation rhinoplasty involves three primary and independent components: (1) avoiding lateral crural resection, (2) subperichondral dissection, and (3) en bloc lowering of the dorsum (dorsal preservation rhinoplasty [DPR]).[1,3–5] DPR has gained particular interest among rhinoplasty surgeons, both clinically and academically, over the course of the last 4 years. It should be emphasized that although dorsal preservation is not a new concept, the recent promotion of this ideology has led to valuable analysis and technical modifications.

HISTORICAL CONTEXT

A detailed history of DPR has been described elsewhere.[6] The earliest description in 1899 by J. Goodale involved lateral and root osteotomies, along with septal resection, to lower the nasal dorsum as a single unit and eliminate a bony-cartilaginous hump.[7,8] This technique resulted in the displacement of the bony vault into the nasal cavity (medial to the maxilla) and in contemporary DPR is known as the push-down (PD) technique (**Fig. 1**). O. Lothrop, in 1914, added wedge resections at the sidewalls so that the lateral aspects of the bony vault rested on the maxilla rather than being displaced medially to it.[9] This has become known as the let-down (LD) procedure (**Fig. 2**).[10–12] As can be ascertained by descriptions by Goodale and Lothrop, dorsal lowering has two requisites: (1) treatment of the external bony vault and (2) resection and mobilization of the underlying septal support.

The authors have no disclosures
[a] Division of Facial Plastic and Reconstructive Surgery, Department of Otolaryngology, Vanderbilt University Medical Center, Nashville, TN, USA; [b] Division of Facial Plastic and Reconstructive Surgery, Stanford University School of Medicine, 801 Welch Road, Stanford, CA 94304, USA
* Corresponding author.
E-mail address: smost@stanford.edu

Facial Plast Surg Clin N Am 31 (2023) 1–11
https://doi.org/10.1016/j.fsc.2022.08.003

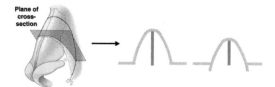

Fig. 1. Push-down (PD) technique. Lateral and transverse (radix) osteotomies combined with septal resection allows for en bloc lowering of the nasal pyramid. The nasal sidewalls are displaced into the nasal cavity.

ANATOMIC AND FUNCTIONAL CONSIDERATIONS

Descriptions of the relationships between the nasal bones, perpendicular plate of the ethmoid (PPE), septal cartilage, and the upper lateral cartilages (ULCs) help elucidate the mechanism and potential benefits of DPR techniques.[4,5,13–15] As a review, the nasal bones fuse with the frontal bone superiorly, giving rise to the externally described radix. A dorsal hump will start at some distance between the radix and the rhinion (bony-cartilaginous junction). The rhinion consists of a nonrigid fusion of perichondrium and periosteum.[16] Therefore, when the dorsum is lowered, there is flexion at this site and elimination of dorsal convexity. The ULCs attach to the midline septum and the undersurface of the nasal bones (overlap of 4–14 mm), giving rise to the medial dorsal and lateral keystone (**Fig. 3**).[16] This lateral junction is semi-rigid and may hinder complete dorsal lowering.

Importantly, the septal cartilage also extends sub-dorsally under the nasal bones (see **Fig. 3**). The most cranial cartilaginous-bony junction has been variably named either the Ethmoidal (E), Keystone (K), or Junctional (J) point.[17] The reported distance between the rhinion and E-point is 4 to 11 mm.[17–21] A dorsal hump therefore largely sits over the cartilaginous septum. As high as 97% of humps may start caudal to the ethmoidal point.[21] These features suggest that when the cartilaginous septum is resected, both the bony and cartilaginous dorsum will descend.

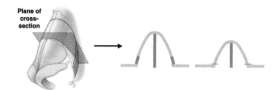

Fig. 2. Let-down (LD) technique. Osteotomies similar to the PD technique are performed with the additional resection of a wedge of bone at the sidewalls. When the dorsum is lowered after septal resection, the nasal sidewalls rest on the maxilla.

The nasal bone profile between the naso-frontal junction and the rhinion may be V-shaped or S-shaped (**Fig. 4**).[22] V-shaped nasal bones have a straight contour along its whole course with an apex at the rhinion. S-shaped nasal bones present a curved contour with the most prominent point (kyphion) present cephalic to the rhinion. These shapes have implications for preservation techniques.

The junction between the ULC and nasal septum contributes to the internal nasal valve (INV). Preservation techniques avoid disruption and the need to reconstruct this anatomically sensitive area. However, given the fusion of the ULC with the nasal bone, positional changes in the bony vault will be transmitted to the cartilaginous middle vault in DPR. In a radiological analysis of patients undergoing either PD or LD, an improved INV angle was noted.[23] In a cadaveric radiologic study, the INV dimensions/angle did not change in the LD technique or joseph hump resection with appropriate midvault reconstruction, but did decrease with the PD technique.[24] This is attributed to the medialization of the nasal sidewall into the nasal cavity with the PD technique. The PD technique can be performed with a lateral ostectomy of bone (thinning the lateral nasal wall) to minimize obstructive sequalea.[25]

INDICATIONS FOR DORSAL PRESERVATION RHINOPLASTY

Although the PD or LD techniques are well recognized as treatment strategies for the bony vault, descriptions of surface modifications (±osteotomies) have introduced new partial approaches to DPR. The contemporary definition of DPR does not require preserving the continuity of the bony-cartilaginous dorsum or treating this unit en bloc, thereby expanding DPR indications. Conceptually, two classes of DPR techniques have been forwarded: (1) foundation techniques and (2) surface techniques.[26,27] The foundational techniques involve impaction of the nasal vault using osteotomies (eg, PD or LD). Surface techniques involve superficial modifications of the dorsal hump without impaction or osteotomies and with optional preservation of the bony cap. What remains true of essentially all DPR cases is that the middle vault is preserved. Surface techniques may help convert patients with suboptimal anatomy into appropriate DPR candidates (eg, bony cap resection or contouring the ULC shoulders).

In general, DPR is limited to primary cases, but may be performed secondarily if similar techniques were used primarily.[11,28,29] Patients with

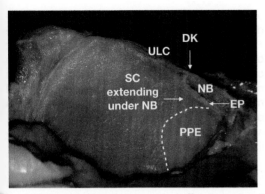

Fig. 3. Dorsal and Keystone anatomy. The dorsal nasal keystone (DK) of the nose consists of the junction of the perpendicular plate of the ethmoid (PPE), nasal bones (NB), septal cartilage (SC), and upper lateral cartilages (ULC). Septal cartilage extends under the nasal bones. Over the dorsum, the perichondrium of the cartilaginous vault and the periosteum of the nasal bones fuse to create a flexible joint.

shorter nasal bones and a larger cartilaginous contribution to the nasal hump are better candidates for DPR.[14] V-shaped nasal bones are better treated with DPR compared with S-shaped bones. The latter group has a higher likelihood of an osseous residual hump without additional contouring maneuvers.[30–32] Patients with deeper nasofrontal angles are at greater risk of a drop in the radix with DPR technqiues.[14] As preservation surgery aims to maintain the shape of the dorsum, inherently deformed bones with irregularities or significant width of either the bones or midvault will result in unsatisfactory outcomes.[14,30,31] It also follows that DPR should be considered in patients with thin skin to minimize risk of visible

dorsal irregularities. As the middle vault cannot be separated from its pyrifom attachments, it will flare as it descends. If there are very wide and prominent ULC shoulders, DPR may predispose to worsening of this appearance. Although deformities of the nasal bones are relative contraindications to DPR, the presence of an axis deviation is not. Asymmetric wedge resections of bone in an LD procedure with more bone removed on the non-deviated side can correct a straight deviation **(Fig. 5)**.[33–35] Alternatively, an LD on the deviated side with a PD on the non-deviated side ("mixdown") can be used.[36] Overlap and suture fixation of subdorsal septum to the lower septum toward the deviated side will help stabilize the corrected position.[37] DPR has been reported to reduce revision rates in males compared with other surgical techniques, potentially due to less risk of feminization.[32] Higher revision rates may be observed in females due to the desire for greater dorsal height reduction.[32]

Although the closed rhinoplasty approach has been used by many preservation experts, DPR can be successfully accomplished with open approaches. The closed approach ensures protection of the dorsal soft tissue and allows for preservation of soft tissue attachments that may be beneficial in the suspension of bone as it descends.[30] The open approach provides greater visualization of the dorsal deformity along its whole course and allows for both osteotomies and fine-tuning of dorsal irregularities with the use of powered instruments.[38] A graded approach to dorsal soft tissue dissection when using an open approach may be considered.[38] In patients with V-shaped nasal bones with well-shaped dorsal

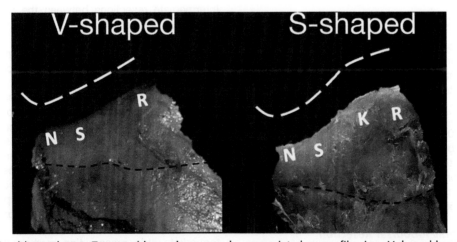

Fig. 4. Nasal bone shapes. Two nasal bone shapes can be appreciated on profile view. V-shaped bones have a straight contour between the radix and the rhinion. S-shaped bones have a curve with a peak (kyphion) between the radix and rhinion.

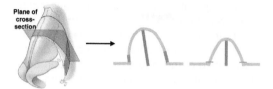

Fig. 5. Deviated nose. Correction of axis deviation in DPR includes asymmetric wedge resections of bone in the LD procedure, with more bone removed on the non-deviated side.

esthetics, preservation of the dorsal soft tissue and ligaments can be performed. In cases that may require osteoplasty (eg, S-shaped bones) or the need to address dorsal irregularities, the dorsal soft tissue is elevated.

Another graded approach in preservation rhinoplasty comes in the form of combination preservation methodology used for the dorsum with structural modifications made to the nasal tip complex.[39,40] This ideology—termed structural preservation—allows for conventional tip modification techniques with an emphasis on preservation and recontouring of the alar cartilage (lateral crural tensioning, cephalic cartilage turn-in flaps, lateral crural struts). In addition, open approaches with the use of tip supporting mechanisms such as septal extension grafts and columellar struts are used as preferred. The dorsum is lowered with preservation techniques. This hybrid approach allows surgeons confident with open structural techniques the opportunity to incorporate preservation techniques into practice. Importantly, the structural and preservation ideologies should not be considered mutually exclusive, but rather concepts that can be fused to produce an esthetically pleasing and stable result.

APPROACHES TO THE NASAL SEPTUM

Perhaps some of the greatest nuances in preservation rhinoplasty relate to the treatment of the nasal septum. Multiple techniques to resect and mobilize the septum had been forwarded during the 1900s by several surgeons.[35,41–50] Further descriptions have been advanced over the course of the last 20 years, resulting in several modifications that can be applied in preservation rhinoplasty. In general, these techniques can be classified by the region of septal cartilage resection: high, mid/intermediate, or low. These are briefly summarized here (**Fig. 6**).

High-Septal/Subdorsal Resection

Following original descriptions by Lothrop, Goodale, and Maurel, contemporary preservation

experts Saban and Gola have championed immediate subdorsal resection of cartilage (see **Fig. 6**A).[7–9,14,35,51,52] Two incisions are made: one immediately under the dorsum, following the contour of the dorsal hump and a second cut more inferiorly corresponding to the desired dorsal height. Intervening cartilage is removed (with possible additional subdorsal ethmoid bone), allowing for the dorsum to be lowered and stabilized with suture fixation.

Low-Septal Excision

Sebileau and Dufourmentel described resection of an inferior strip of bone and cartilage to allow for dorsal height reduction (see **Fig. 6**B).[48] The septum requires stabilization to the maxillary crest. In 1946, M. Cottle performed a modification of the inferior strip with the additional disarticulation of the cartilaginous septum from the ethmoid plate and resection of PPE immediately under the dorsum (see **Fig. 6**C).[49,53] This resulted in a complete vertical split between the bony and cartilaginous septum, with the dorsum being lowered secondary to the high bony and low cartilaginous resection. The Septum Pyramidal Adjustment and Repositioning (SPAR) method described by Dewes similarly involves an inferior removal of cartilage or maxillary crest, a posterior chondrotomy, and resection of a portion of the PPE.[54] The disarticulation of the whole cartilaginous septum through an inferior release are beneficial in cases of deviated septal pathology as it allows complete repositioning.[38] However, this also requires adequate anchoring of the cartilage to the maxillary crest.

Mid-Septal/Intermediate Excision

Intermediate resections between the immediate subdorsal and inferior portions of the septum have been the most variably described. In these methods, some cartilage remains immediately below the dorsum and this can be anchored to lower cartilage with suture techniques, thereby better stabilizing the dorsal position. Ishida and colleagues[50] described a mid-septal strip excision that extends from the caudal border of the septum to the PPE at the level of the transverse osteotomy (see **Fig. 6**D). Although nasal bones were resected/treated independently from the middle vault in this technique (thereby differing from traditional DPR techniques), the location of septal cartilage excision is an important modification. Neves and colleagues[55] have similarly reported on an intermediate strip preservation method (Vitruvian Man Split maneuver) in which the addition of a vertical chondrotomy at the prominent point of the

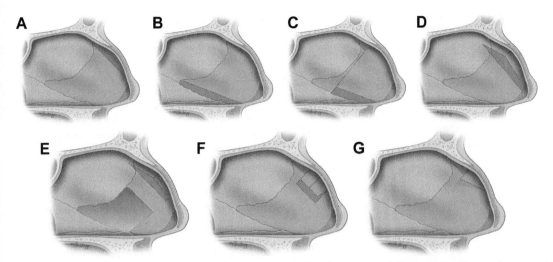

Fig. 6. Approaches to the septum in dorsal preservation rhinoplasty. Dotted lines represent septal cuts and shaded gray areas representing resected segments of cartilage. (*A*) Subdorsal resection: An incision is made immediately under the dorsum, following the contour of the dorsal hump. A second cut below this level dictates the amount of cartilage resected. (*B*) Inferior strip: A segment of inferior cartilage at the maxillary crest is resected. (*C*) Cottle/SPAR method: A segment of ethmoid bone is resected superiorly and cartilage is excised inferiorly at the maxillary crest. The cartilaginous septum is separated from the ethmoid plate. (*D*) Intermediate septal resection: Septal strip excision is performed closer to the mid-aspect of the cartilaginous septum. A vertical chondrotomy (Vitruvian method) at the prominent point of the hump facilitates dorsal flexion. (*E*) Modified subdorsal strip method (MSSM): A 3–5 mm subdorsal strut of cartilage is preserved with cuts made posterior to the anterior septal angle, thereby allowing for the preservation of a caudal strut. Vertical incisions can be made into the subdorsal cartilage to facilitate flexion. Additional cartilage is resected inferiorly as needed for grafting/deviation as needed. This results in a remaining "T" strut of cartilage. (*F*) Split tetris concept: A 5–8-mm "tetris block" is designed in the septum. A segment of cartilage is resected inferior to this and posterior to this (subdorsally). An incision into the tetris block at its mid-aspect helps facilitate dorsal flexion. (*G*) Kovacevic technique: A high posterior bone resection is performed and a triangular cartilaginous wedge is maintained anteriorly. Under this, cartilage is not resected but instead the triangular wedge overlaps and is fixated to the lower septum.

hump allows for better dorsal flexion. This technique can be applied to several intermediate septal resection techniques that preserve a segment of subdorsal cartilage.

Most have reported on a modified subdorsal strip method (MSSM) in which the septal resection is performed higher than the mid-septal approach described by Ishida (leaving a 5 mm subdorsal strut) (see **Fig. 6**E).[28,56] In addition, the septal resections are not carried into the caudal septum and instead start posterior to the anterior septal angle. Inferior cartilage can be removed for grafting purposes. This leaves a "T" strut of cartilage that involves the caudal septum and an intact mid-septal segment. The caudal septum can either be trimmed secondarily or left in its original location to allow for attachment of the tripod complex.

The Split Tetris Concept represents another modification of the intermediate septal resection (see **Fig. 6**F).[37,57] A 5-8-mm subdorsal "tetris block" is designed in the septum between the caudal edge of the ULCs (W point) and the apex of the dorsal hump. Under this, a trapezoid segment of cartilage is excised. Similar to other techniques, the amount of this excision corresponds to the desired dorsal height reduction. To facilitate the lowering process, a posterior triangular wedge of subdorsal cartilage and sometimes bone is also resected to the level of the transverse osteotomy. The combined posterior high bone resection and anterior cartilaginous septal resection shares features with the Cottle method. To allow room for the anterior movement with flexion of the dorsum, an anterior segment of the tetris block may have to be resected. Kovacevic has described a similar modification to the Cottle technique (Subdorsal Z flap; see **Fig. 6**G).[4,58–61] Rather than a rectangular subdorsal block, a triangular cartilaginous wedge is maintained. In this technique, whereas a subdorsal bony keel is removed posterior to the cartilaginous triangular wedge, a segment of cartilage is not resected below it. Instead, this subdorsal segment of cartilage is overlapped and suture fixated to the inferior cartilage. The preservation of some amount of subdorsal cartilage is thought to limit the risk of scar contracture that can deform the middle vault over time.[58]

APPROACHES TO THE OSSEO-CARTILAGINOUS COMPLEX

As aforementioned, although the PD and LD techniques have traditionally been the hallmark of preservation rhinoplasty, modifications that may not treat the whole bony-cartilaginous vault en bloc have been incorporated into preservation idealogy.[59] In cases with extremely kyphotic humps, the use of disarticulation techniques in which the bony dorsum and middle vault are treated independently may use preservation techniques where complete structural approaches would have otherwise been used.[32]

For example, Ishida and colleagues[50] describe a mid-septal cartilage resection with lowering and preservation of the midvault. However, the nasal bones are disarticulated from the ULC, and the osseous hump is treated independently with the use of osteotomes or rasps. Ozturk has described a similar approach in which a subdorsal strip is instead resected to lower the midvault.[62] No osteotomies are performed. These techniques may only be useful in the setting of smaller dorsal humps and may require grafting at the keystone.

A modification of these techniques aims to preserve the continuity between the bony cap and cartilaginous dorsum (cartilage PD technique with bony cap preservation).[63] Separation of the ULCs from the nasal bones as well as disarticulation of the whole septal bony-cartilaginous junction are performed. After resection of septal cartilage, osteotomies along the dorsal esthetic lines that meet in the midline are performed. These osteotomies encompass the bony cap and result in a mobile complex involving the septum and dorsum (including the bony cap), which allows for lowering of a dorsal hump. The remaining bony vault is then contoured as necessary with the use of lateral osteotomies to medialize the nasal bones. This strategy preserves the dorsal cartilage-bony junction and allows for preservation methods to be applied in the setting of larger humps or more distorted bony architecture.

The Spare Roof Technique described by Ferriera and colleagues[64] represents another middle third preservation technique in which the dorsum is lowered via subdorsal cartilage resection. The bony nasal vault is managed with separation of the pyriform aperture ligaments, an ostectomy of the caudal aspect of nasal bones (to expose the cephalic aspect of the ULCs), and medial and lateral osteotomies to close the open bony roof.

A modified dorsal split preservation technique described by Robotti and colleagues[65] can be applied in patients with very small bony humps. In this method, the bony hump is minimally rasped and the continuity of the nasal bones to the cartilaginous dorsum is preserved. In this method, unlike the previously described techniques, the ULCs are separated from the cartilaginous septum. This results in a septal "T" component which includes the upper aspect of the septum and its horizontally flared edges. The combination of subdorsal cartilage resection with a traditional PD/LD technique is performed to lower the dorsum. The septal "T" is then re-sutured to the underlying septum and the ULCs.

In another modified preservation technique (Dorsal Roof Technique), Tas describes the preservation of the dorsal bony-cartilaginous junction, but disarticulation of the ULCs from the septum.[66] Medial osteotomies (at the dorsal esthetic lines) and a radix osteotomy are performed such that the whole bony-cartilaginous dorsum descends into the nose en bloc. Lateral and transverse osteotomies are then performed to narrow the dorsum and eliminate the space created by descent of the mid aspect of the bony vault. The ULCs are then sutured to the midline.

DORSAL PRESERVATION OUTCOMES

As DPR techniques continue to evolve and their use becomes more prevalent, critical analysis of long-term outcomes will become imperative. Proponents of dorsal preservation techniques cite theoretic benefits that stem from preservation of the keystone area, the ULC attachment to the septum, and the INV. As the native attachments of the dorsum are not violated, DPR should yield superior esthetic outcomes with maintenance of dorsal esthetic lines and minimization of surface irregularities (**Fig. 7**).[28,67] Functional benefits compared with conventional hump reduction techniques with appropriate midvault reconstruction may not be as convincing, and studies comparing outcomes with joseph hump reduction are limited at present.[68]

Nonetheless, multiple authors have reported on positive outcomes with PD and LD DPR techniques. In a series of 320 patients undergoing subdorsal resection DPR, Saban and colleagues[14] have reported good success. Of 30 patients given the Nasal Obstruction Symptom Evaluation (NOSE) questionnaire, 90% of patients reported improvements. Although measures are not reported, similar positive results have been described by Gola (n = 1000) and Tuncel and Aydogdu (n = 520).[29,69] In 58 patients undergoing either PD or LD DPR and completing the rhinoplasty outcomes evaluation (ROE), long term patient satisfaction and quality of life was improved.[70] In a group undergoing the MSSM

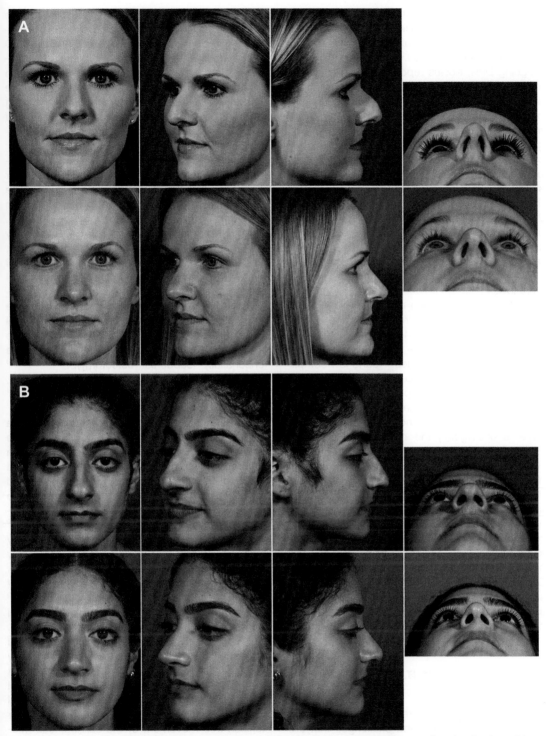

Fig. 7. Structural-preservation rhinoplasty patient examples. (*A*) This patient underwent dorsal reduction with os-seocartilaginous dorsal preservation (let-down, modified subdorsal strip method, two suture fixation, pyriform ligament release) with tongue-in-groove and alar-spanning sutures used to support and adjust the nasal tip po-sition. Pre- and postoperative 18-month photos are shown here. (*B*) This patient underwent dorsal reduction with osseocartilaginous dorsal preservation similar to the patient in A. The nasal tip was managed with minimal ce-phalic trims, intradomal, and interdomal sutures, tongue-in-groove/alar-spanning sutures, and a supratip morsel-ized cartilage graft. Pre- and postoperative 6-month photos are shown here.

method, improved patient postoperative Standardized Cosmesis and Health Nasal Outcomes Survey scores and visual analog scale (VAS) scores have been reported.[28,56] Of 31 patients undergoing DPR, Kosins reports success at 1 year follow up (20% required radix grafts to maintain radix position and 10%, had a very mild residual hump).[3] In 153 patients undergoing the SPAR method, Atolini and colleagues[71] similarly report good outcomes with 13 requiring revisions for small residual humps. Kovacevic has also reported success in 205 patients undergoing the subdorsal triangular resection method with less than 10% revision rates.[61] In a meta-analysis of 22 studies representing a cohort of 5660 patients undergoing a variety of DPR techniques, postoperative hump recurrence rates (4.18%), rates of revision surgery (3.48%), postoperative nasal deviation (1.13%) and rates of infection (1.89%) were low.[72]

Success has also been reported in DPR techniques with modified approaches to the osseocartilaginous complex. In 48 patients undergoing the cartilage PD technique with bony cap preservation, Ishida and colleagues[63] found low complication rates: 1 had displacement of the bony cap and 1 experienced a hump recurrence. In 44 patients undergoing the Dorsal Roof technique, positive ROE results were noted at 1 year.[66] 62 patients undergoing the modified cartilaginous PD maneuver by Ozturk also reported positive ROE outcomes.[62] In 41 patients undergoing the dorsal split preservation technique and 120 patients undergoing mid-septal cartilage resection favorable outcomes have been reported.[50,65] An analysis of 1 year postoperative outcomes in 100 patients who underwent the spare roof technique showed improved functional and esthetic VAS scores as well as Utrecht Questionnaire for Outcome Assessment in Esthetic Rhinoplasty scores.[73] In a randomized prospective study (n = 250) comparing this technique to component dorsal hump reduction, VAS scores were superior in the former group.[74]

CHALLENGES AND LIMITATIONS OF DORSAL PRESERVATION

Despite the benefits of preservation techniques, there are complications and challenges that are unique to DPR. One of the most cited concerns relates to recurrence of a dorsal hump, with rates ranging between 3% and 12%.[3,14,29,50,71,75] The maximal tension at the dorsum will exist at the apex of the dorsal hump. Therefore, the risk of hump recurrence is greater with increased prominence of the hump apex and in S shaped nasal

bones. Methods to minimize hump recurrence may include (1) scoring/incising subdorsal cartilage to maximize cartilage flexion, (2) using LD preferentially over the PD, (3) multi-site suture fixation oriented in both cranio-caudal and posterior-anterior dimensions, (4) additional bone contouring in kyphotic humps, and (5) performing a lateral keystone dissection with separation of the ULCs from the nasal bones (ballerina maneuver/lateral wall split maneuver).[29,37,75,76]

There is also risk of excessive inferior displacement of the upper nasal vault, resulting in a lower than desired dorsal height and/or a step-off at the radix. Unless the patient has a high radix, flexion rather than descent is needed at this location. Methods to minimize excessive descent may include (1) conservative resection of septal bone, (2) a longitudinal cut into rather than resection of the bony septum (3) a triangular shaped subdorsal wedge resection rather than a rectangle, (4) preservation of periosteum and soft tissue over the midline dorsum/radix to provide support at the level of the transverse osteotomy, and (5) transverse osteotomy made obliquely and potentially made endonasally (subdorsal osteotomy).[19,27,28,30,57,58] Radix grafting may be necessary for camouflage, as was reported in 20% of the patients in Kosins' study.[3]

Although radiographic studies have confirmed a safe distance between the cribiform plate and the location of the transverse osteotomy site, there is a theoretic risk of propagating forces inferiorly and posteriorly, disruption of the cribriform plate, and a CSF leak.[19,20,58] Carefully oriented and complete osteotomies, in addition to the use of piezo ultrasonic instruments can help mitigate this risk.[76–79] In addition, the ethmoid bone should be carefully resected/incised to the level of the osteotomy before the transverse osteotomy is made.

Supratip saddling is a potential complication of DPR, particularly in low septal approaches.[30] This may be related to the persistence of a dorsal convexity (with a drop in the supratip region), greater difficulty in controlling septal height, and inadequate fixation of the septum to the maxillary crest. Another stigmata involves midvault widening.[30] Although this may have functional benefits, it can be esthetically displeasing. Lateral keystone disarticulation can release the ULC for tension-free movement of the cartilaginous midvault and help prevent flaring in this region.

SUMMARY

DPR is likely to continue to evolve and become more widely adopted into clinical practice. This ideology emphasizes an appreciation for nasal anatomy, along with esthetic and functional implications of disrupting this anatomy. Although alar preservation has been promoted for the last two decades in structural rhinoplasty, there is a recognized value in the incorporation of dorsal preservation into similar practice. This fusion, structural preservation, affords the rhinoplasty surgeon a large tool-set to maximize esthetic and functional outcomes. Understanding the foundations of DPR—namely septal resection and the osseo-cartilaginous mobilization—in addition to the anatomic nuances, modifications, and indications as are reviewed here will facilitate the implementation of these techniques into clinical practice. In the process, the critical analysis of long-term outcomes and limitations, particularly as they compare to conventional hump resection, should be pursued.

CLINICS CARE POINTS

- Open structural tip methods can be combined with dorsal preservation techniques

- Although preservation techniques have garnered significant attention secondary to esthetic benefits, conventional hump resection techniques with appropriate midvault reconstruction may yield equivalent functional outcomes

- Not all patients are candidates for preservation rhinoplasty and an understanding of best indications (eg, limited kyphosis and pleasing preoperative dorsal architecture) will maximize positive outcomes and minimize complications

- Different modifications in septal and osseo-cartilaginous DPR approaches are available to the rhinoplasty surgeon—each of which has been shown to yield positive outcomes

- Minimizing stigmata of preservation rhinoplasty including hump recurrence, mid-vault widening, and radix step offs require an understanding of anatomic and technical nuances

REFERENCES

1. Daniel RK. The Preservation Rhinoplasty: A New Rhinoplasty Revolution. Aesthet Surg J 2018;38(2): 228–9.

2. Patel PN, Kandathil CK, Buba CM, et al. Global Practice Patterns of Dorsal Preservation Rhinoplasty. Facial Plast Surg Aesthet Med 2021. https://doi.org/10.1089/fpsam.2021.0055.

3. Kosins AM, Daniel RK. Decision Making in Preservation Rhinoplasty: A 100 Case Series With One-Year Follow-Up. Aesthet Surg J 2020;40(1):34–48.

4. Çakır B, Saban Y, Daniel RK, et al. Preservation rhinoplasty Book. Istanbul, Turkey: Septum Publishing; 2018.

5. Daniel RK, Palhazi P. The Nasal Ligaments and Tip Support in Rhinoplasty: An Anatomical Study. Aesthet Surg J 2018;38(4):357–68.

6. Kern EB. History of Dorsal Preservation Surgery: Seeking Our Historical Godfather(s) for the "Push Down" and "Let Down" Operations. Facial Plast Surg Clin North Am 2021;29(1):1–14.

7. Goodale JL. A New Method for the Operative Correction of Exaggerated Roman Nose. Boston Med Surg J 1899;140:112.

8. Goodale JL. The Correction of Old Lateral Displacements of the Nasal Bones. Boston Med Surg J 1901; 145:538–9.

9. Lothrop O. An operation for correcting the aquiline nasal deformity; the use of new instrument; report of a case. Boston Med Surg J 1914;170: 835–7.

10. FL. U. Let down technique. Available at: https://www.rhinoplastyarchive.com/articles/let-down-technique. Accessed December 12, 2019.

11. Montes-Bracchini JJ. Nasal Profile Hump Reduction Using the Let-Down Technique. Facial Plast Surg 2019;35(5):486–91.

12. Montes-Bracchini JJ. Preservation Rhinoplasty (Let-Down Technique) for Endonasal Dorsal Reduction. Facial Plast Surg Clin North Am 2021; 29(1):59–66.

13. Cakir B, Oreroglu AR, Dogan T, et al. A complete subperichondrial dissection technique for rhinoplasty with management of the nasal ligaments. Aesthet Surg J 2012;32(5):564–74.

14. Saban Y, Daniel RK, Polselli R, et al. Dorsal Preservation: The Push Down Technique Reassessed. Aesthet Surg J 2018;38(2):117–31.

15. Abdelwahab M, Patel PN. Conventional Resection Versus Preservation of the Nasal Dorsum and Ligaments: An Anatomic Perspective and Review of the Literature. Facial Plast Surg Clin North Am 2021; 29(1):15–28.

16. Palhazi P, Daniel RK, Kosins AM. The osseocartilaginous vault of the nose: anatomy and surgical observations. Aesthet Surg J 2015;35(3):242–51.

17. Ferreira MG, Dias DR, Cardoso L, et al. Dorsal Hump Reduction Based on the New Ethmoidal Point Classification: A Clinical and Radiological Study of the Keystone Area in 138 Patients. Aesthet Surg J 2020;40(9):950–9.

18. Eravci FC, Ozer H, Arbag H, et al. Computed Tomography Analysis of Nasal Anatomy in Dorsal Preservation Rhinoplasty. Aesthet Surg J 2022;42(3): 249–56.

19. Sadri A, East C, Badia L, et al. Dorsal Preservation Rhinoplasty: Core Beam Computed Tomography Analysis of the Nasal Vault, Septum, and Skull Base-Its Role in Surgical Planning. Facial Plast Surg 2020;36(3):329–34.

20. Demirel O, Atesci MS. Preservation Rhinoplasty: Assessment of Anatomical Safe Boundaries on Computed Tomography. J Craniofac Surg 2022; 33(2):570–4.

21. Rodrigues Dias D, Cardoso L, Santos M, et al. The Caucasian Hump: Radiologic Study of the Osteocartilaginous Vault versus Surface Anatomy. Clinical Implications in Structured and Preservation Rhinoplasty. Plast Reconstr Surg 2021;148(3):523–31.

22. Lazovic GD, Daniel RK, Janosevic LB, et al. Rhinoplasty: the nasal bones - anatomy and analysis. Aesthet Surg J 2015;35(3):255–63.

23. Stergiou G, Fortuny CG, Schweiger A, et al. A multivariate analysis after preservation rhinoplasty (PR) - a prospective study. J Plast Reconstr Aesthet Surg 2022;75(1):369–73.

24. Abdelwahab MA, Neves CA, Patel PN, et al. Impact of Dorsal Preservation Rhinoplasty Versus Dorsal Hump Resection on the Internal Nasal Valve: a Quantitative Radiological Study. Aesthet Plast Surg 2020;44(3):879–87.

25. Ozturk G. Push down technique with ostectomy. Ann Chir Plast Esthet 2020.

26. Goncalves Ferreira M, Toriumi DM. A Practical Classification System for Dorsal Preservation Rhinoplasty Techniques. Facial Plast Surg Aesthet Med 2021; 23(3):153–5.

27. Ferreira MG, Santos M, Dias D. Subdorsal Osteotomy and Complete Dorsal Preservation - A New Paradigm in Preservation Rhinoplasty? Laryngoscope 2022;132(4):769–71.

28. Patel PN, Abdelwahab M, Most SP. A Review and Modification of Dorsal Preservation Rhinoplasty Techniques. Facial Plast Surg Aesthet Med 2020; 22(2):71–9.

29. Tuncel U, Aydogdu O. The Probable Reasons for Dorsal Hump Problems following Let-Down/Push-Down Rhinoplasty and Solution Proposals. Plast Reconstr Surg 2019;144(3):378e–85e.

30. Neves JC, Arancibia-Tagle D. Avoiding Esthetic Drawbacks and Stigmata in Dorsal Line Preservation Rhinoplasty. Facial Plast Surg 2021;37(1): 65–75.

31. Ferraz MBJ, Sella GCP. Indications for Preservation Rhinoplasty: Avoiding Complications. Facial Plast Surg 2021;37(1):45–52.

32. Saban Y, de Salvador S. Guidelines for Dorsum Preservation in Primary Rhinoplasty. Facial Plast Surg 2021;37(1):53–64.

33. Ozucer B, Cam OH. The Effectiveness of Asymmetric Dorsal Preservation for Correction of I-Shaped Crooked Nose Deformity in Comparison to Conventional Technique. Facial Plast Surg Aesthet Med 2020;22(4):286–93.

34. East C. Preservation Rhinoplasty and the Crooked Nose. Facial Plast Surg Clin North Am 2021;29(1): 123–30.

35. Maurel G. Chirurgie maxilla-faciale. Paris: Le François; 1940. p. 1127–33.

36. Ozturk G. Hybrid Preservation Rhinoplasty: Combining Mix-Down and Semi Let-Push Down Techniques. J Craniofac Surg 2022. https://doi.org/10.1097/SCS.0000000000008553.

37. Neves JC, Tagle DA, Dewes W, et al. A Segmental Approach in Dorsal Preservation Rhinoplasty: The Tetris Concept. Facial Plast Surg Clin North Am 2021;29(1):85–99.

38. Goksel A, Saban Y, Tran KN. Biomechanical Nasal Anatomy Applied to Open Preservation Rhinoplasty. Facial Plast Surg 2021;37(1):12–21.

39. Toriumi DM, Kovacevic M, Kosins AM. Structural Preservation Rhinoplasty: A Hybrid Approach. Plast Reconstr Surg 2022. https://doi.org/10.1097/PRS.0000000000009063.

40. Patel PN, Most SP. Combining Open Structural and Dorsal Preservation Rhinoplasty. Clin Plast Surg 2022;49(1):97–109.

41. Huizing EH. Push-down of the external nasal pyramid by resection of wedges. Rhinology 1975;13(4): 185–90.

42. Wayoff M, Perrin C. [Global mobilization of the nasal pyramid according to Cottle's technic: its possibilities in functional nose surgery]. Acta Otorhinolaryngol Belg 1968;22(6):675–80. Mobilisation globale de la pyramide nasale selon Cottle: ses possibilites dans la chirurgie fonctionnelle du nez.

43. Pirsig W, Konigs D. Wedge resection in rhinosurgery: a review of the literature and long-term results in a hundred cases. Rhinology 1988;26(2):77–88.

44. Willemot J, Vrebos J, Pollet J, et al. [Plastic surgery and otorhinolaryngology]. Acta Otorhinolaryngol Belg 1967;21(5):463–732.

45. Barelli PA. Long term evaluation of "push down" procedures. Rhinology 1975;13(1):25–32.

46. Drumheller GW. The push down operation and septal surgery. Esthetic Plastic surgery: rhinoplasty. Boston, MA: Little, Brown, and Company; 1973.

47. Hinderer KH. Fundamentals of anatomy and surgery of the nose. Birmingham, AL: Aesculapius Publishing Co; 1971.

48. P S, L D. Correction chirurgicale des difformités congénitales et acquises de la pyramide nasale. Paris: Arnette; 1926. p. 104–5.

49. Cottle MH, Loring RM. Corrective surgery of the external nasal pyramid and the nasal septum for restoration of normal physiology. Ill Med J 1946;90: 119–35.

50. Ishida J, Ishida LC, Ishida LH, et al. Treatment of the nasal hump with preservation of the cartilaginous

framework. Plast Reconstr Surg 1999;103(6): 1729–33 [discussion: 1734–5].

51. Gola R, Nerini A, Laurent-Fyon C, et al. [Conservative rhinoplasty of the nasal canopy]. Ann Chir Plast Esthet 1989;34(6):465–75. Rhinoplastie conservatrice de l'auvent nasal.

52. Saban Y, Braccini F, Polselli R. [Rhinoplasty: morphodynamic anatomy of rhinoplasty. Interest of conservative rhinoplasty]. Rev Laryngol Otol Rhinol (Bord) 2006;127(1–2):15–22. La rhinoplastie : anatomie morpho-dynamique de la rhinoplastie. Interet de la rhinoplastie "conservatrice.

53. Friedman O, Ulloa FL, Kern EB. Preservation Rhinoplasty: The Endonasal Cottle Push-Down/Let-Down Approach. Facial Plast Surg Clin North Am 2021; 29(1):67–75.

54. Ferraz M, Zappelini CEM, Carvalho GM, et al. Cirurgia conservadora do dorso nasal – a filosofia do reposicionamento e ajuste do septo piramidal (S.P.A.R.). Rev Bras Cir Cabeça Pescoço 2013;42:124–30.

55. Neves JC, Arancibia Tagle D, Dewes W, et al. The split preservation rhinoplasty: "the Vitruvian Man split maneuver". Eur J Plast Surg volume 2020;43:323–33.

56. Patel PN, Abdelwahab M, Most SP. Dorsal Preservation Rhinoplasty: Method and Outcomes of the Modified Subdorsal Strip Method. Facial Plast Surg Clin North Am 2021;29(1):29–37.

57. Neves JC, Arancibia Tagle D, Dewes W, et al. The Segmental Preservation Rhinoplasty: The Split Tetris Concept. Facial Plast Surg 2020. https://doi.org/10.1055/s-0040-1714672.

58. Toriumi DM, Kovacevic M. Dorsal Preservation Rhinoplasty: Measures to Prevent Suboptimal Outcomes. Facial Plast Surg Clin North Am 2021; 29(1):141–53.

59. Kosins AM. Expanding Indications for Dorsal Preservation Rhinoplasty With Cartilage Conversion Techniques. Aesthet Surg J 2020. https://doi.org/10.1093/asj/sjaa071.

60. Kovacevic M, Veit JA, Toriumi DM. Subdorsal Z-flap: a modification of the Cottle technique in dorsal preservation rhinoplasty. Curr Opin Otolaryngol Head Neck Surg 2021;29(4):244–51.

61. Kovacevic M, Buttler E, Haack S, et al. [Dorsal preservation septorhinoplasty]. HNO 2020. https://doi.org/10.1007/s00106-020-00949-3. Die nasenruckenerhaltende "Dorsal-Preservation"-Septorhinoplastik.

62. Ozturk G. Push-Down Technique Without Osteotomy: A New Approach. Aesthet Plast Surg 2020; 44(3):891–901.

63. Ishida LC, Ishida J, Ishida LH, et al. Nasal Hump Treatment With Cartilaginous Push-Down and Preservation of the Bony Cap. Aesthet Surg J 2020; 40(11):1168–78.

64. Ferreira MG, Monteiro D, Reis C, et al. Spare Roof Technique: A Middle Third New Technique. Facial Plast Surg 2016;32(1):111–6.

65. Robotti E, Chauke-Malinga NY, Leone F. A Modified Dorsal Split Preservation Technique for Nasal Humps with Minor Bony Component: A Preliminary Report. Aesthet Plast Surg 2019;43(5):1257–68.

66. Tas S. Dorsal Roof Technique for Dorsum Preservation in Rhinoplasty. Aesthet Surg J 2020;40(3): 263–75.

67. Patel PN, Abdelwahab M, Most SP. Combined Functional and Preservation Rhinoplasty. Facial Plast Surg Clin North Am 2021;29(1):113–21.

68. Levin M, Ziai H, Roskies M. Patient Satisfaction following Structural versus Preservation Rhinoplasty: A Systematic Review. Facial Plast Surg 2020. https://doi.org/10.1055/s-0040-1714268.

69. Gola R. Functional and esthetic rhinoplasty. Aesthet Plast Surg 2003;27(5):390–6.

70. Stergiou G, Schweigler A, Finocchi V, et al. Quality of Life (QoL) and Outcome After Preservation Rhinoplasty (PR) Using the Rhinoplasty Outcome Evaluation (ROE) Questionnaire-A Prospective Observational Single-Centre Study. Aesthet Plast Surg 2022. https://doi.org/10.1007/s00266-022-02773-2.

71. Atolini NJ, Lunelli V, Lang GP, et al. Septum pyramidal adjustment and repositioning - a conservative and effective rhinoplasty technique. Braz J Otorhinolaryngol 2019;85(2):176–82.

72. Tham T, Bhuiya S, Wong A, et al. Clinical Outcomes in Dorsal Preservation Rhinoplasty: A Meta-Analysis. Facial Plast Surg Aesthet Med 2022. https://doi.org/10.1089/fpsam.2021.0312.

73. Santos M, Rego AR, Coutinho M, et al. Spare roof technique in reduction rhinoplasty: Prospective study of the first one hundred patients. Laryngoscope 2019;129(12):2702–6.

74. Ferreira MG, Santos M, Carmo DOE, et al. Spare Roof Technique Versus Component Dorsal Hump Reduction: A Randomized Prospective Study in 250 Primary Rhinoplasties, Esthetic and Functional Outcomes. Aesthet Surg J 2020. https://doi.org/10.1093/asj/sjaa221.

75. Tuncel U, Aydogdu IO, Kurt A. Reducing Dorsal Hump Recurrence Following Push Down-Let Down Rhinoplasty. Aesthet Surg J 2020. https://doi.org/10.1093/asj/sjaa145.

76. Goksel A, Saban Y. Open Piezo Preservation Rhinoplasty: A Case Report of the New Rhinoplasty Approach. Facial Plast Surg 2019;35(1):113–8.

77. Goksel A, Patel PN, Most SP. Piezoelectric Osteotomies in Dorsal Preservation Rhinoplasty. Facial Plast Surg Clin North Am 2021;29(1):77–84.

78. Almazov I, Rovira RV, Farhadov V. Closed Piezo Preservation Rhinoplasty. Aesthet Plast Surg 2022. https://doi.org/10.1007/s00266-021-02751-0.

79. Taglialatela Scafati S, Regalado-Briz A. Piezo-Assisted Dorsal Preservation in Rhinoplasty: When and Why. Aesthet Plast Surg 2021. https://doi.org/10.1007/s00266-021-02261-z.

Long-Term Follow-Up with Dorsal Preservation Rhinoplasty

Masoud Saman, MD[a],*, Yves Saban, MD[b]

KEYWORDS

- Preservation rhinoplasty ● Dorsal preservation ● Rhinoplasty complications
- Dorsal hump recurrence ● Push down procedure ● Axis deviation ● Revision rhinoplasty

KEY POINTS

- There has been a rapid resurgence of interest in dorsal preservation in recent years.
- Long-term results for dorsal preservation techniques have not been previously published.
- The most common postoperative complication following dorsal preservation is related to persistence or recurrence of the dorsal hump and is amenable to relatively simple in-office rasping.
- Major complications such as polly beak deformity, open roof deformity, and valve stenosis and collapse are not commonly seen in dorsal preservation.
- Revisionary surgery following dorsal preservation is simpler and quicker relative to structural rhinoplasty, seldom if ever, requiring rib or auricular cartilage grafting.
- Dorsal preservation results are stable overtime with high satisfaction rate for surgeon and patients alike.

BACKGROUND

Although dorsal preservation (DP) in rhinoplasty is not a novel concept, there has been a resurgence of interest in this approach and technique since Saban's landmark 2018 article, Dorsal Preservation: The Push Down Technique Reassessed.[1] An increasing number of teaching programs are gradually including formal training in preservation rhinoplasty (PR); however, most of the rhinoplasty surgeons currently performing DP are self-taught and find their formal training centered on structural rhinoplasty. The rapid growth in interest and performance of DP and scarcity of standardized training programs have naturally led to confusion in nomenclature, patient selection criteria, as well as in clinical and surgical decision-making among rhinoplasty surgeons. In view of this lack of consensus, several thought-leaders have provided practical contributions to the PR rhinoplasty literature in recent years. In 2021, Saban furnished a systematic guideline in patient selection in PR.[2] Subsequently, Ferreira and Toriumi provided a classification to systematize PR and to organize thoughts in regard to this resurging hot concept in rhinoplasty.[3] In this article, the authors aim to further contribute to PR literature by providing long-term follow-up with DP, specifically presenting data related to superior strip DP functional and esthetic complications, followed by a detailed analysis of the same. Our data do not include other DP techniques such as Cottle or other related techniques (SPQR, Tetris, and so forth)

BRIEF HISTORY OF DORSAL PRESERVATION

Although classical Jacques Joseph dorsal hump excision has been the mainstay rhinoplasty teaching for the past several decades, DP is not a novel concept. Goodale is credited with the first description dorsal reduction with excision in 1898.[4] This was then followed by Lothrop in

[a] Saman Facial Plastic Surgery, PLLC, 240 Central Park South, New York, NY 10025, USA; [b] Private Practice, 31 Avenue Jean Medecin, Nice 06000, France
* Corresponding author.
E-mail address: msaman309@gmail.com

Facial Plast Surg Clin N Am 31 (2023) 13–24
https://doi.org/10.1016/j.fsc.2022.08.004
1064-7406/23/© 2022 Elsevier Inc. All rights reserved.

Boston describing the first let down operation (LDO) in 1914.[5] Subsequently Sebileau and Dufourmentel further contributed to LDO in 1926.[6] Maurel reported his experience with the Lothrop technique in 1940,[7] using a high septal resection followed by lateral osteotomy of the frontal processes of the maxilla.

Cottle's description of the *push down technique* (PDO) in 1946[8] preserved nasal dorsal contiguity by impaction of the osteocartilaginous hump around the keystone point while leaving the keystone point untouched. Although his septal technique was difficult to master for most surgeons, the concept of PDO had the advantage of keeping the upper lateral cartilages (ULCs) with the nasal bone and thus preventing valve stenosis, often seen with humpectomy techniques. As such, Cottle's PDO technique became popular in the 1960s.

In 1989, Gola simplified the septal portion of Cottle's PDO simply by removing a strip of septal cartilage just below the nasal dorsum.[9] Although Saban used the Cottle technique with excellent results, in the early 1990s he transitioned from Cottle PDO technique to superior septal strip; an approach that he has championed ever since with now over 30 years of experience.

OPERATIVE ANATOMY AND RATIONALE

A strong understanding of nasal anatomy is crucial in the learning and application of DP techniques. Although a comprehensive discussion of nasal anatomy and surgical anatomy pertinent to DP is beyond the scope of this article, the authors believe a brief refresher on nasal dorsal analysis related to soft tissues, cartilage and bony anatomy may be helpful in better understanding some of the most common dorsal complications related to DP.

- Segmental Analysis of Nasal Dorsum
  - The relationship between three dorsal segments, namely the radix, keystone area (KA), and supratip is crucial in dorsal analysis. The radix is a depression at the root of the nose. It defines the root of the nose and its origin from the glabella. The radix is centered over the nasion and involves four different bones. Inferiorly, the radix spans from the nasion to the level of a horizontal line passing through medial canthi, and superiorly from the nasion for the same distance (**Fig. 1**) Cottle coined the term KA in 1954[10] to denote the junction between the nasal bones and the ULC. KA is covered by thin, mostly aponeurotic soft tissue envelope (STE). Dorsally, the overlap of the nasal bones over the cartilaginous septum

forms a chondro-osseous joint. This area is termed the dorsal key stone area (DKA).[11] The W-point denotes the most caudal junction of the ULC and the septum. The area of the septum extending from the W-area to the anterior septal angle (ASA) corresponds to the supratip (W-ASA segment) (**Fig. 1**).

Dorsal analysis therefore may represent several variations of the segments discussed above. The radix may be low, normal, or high. Similarly, KA may straight or convex. The height of KA, which denotes the height of dorsal convexity, is paramount in the decision-making for the technique and approach. The supratip segment may be straight or convex. The STE is quite thick in this region mostly due to SMAS extensions and deep Pitanguy ligament.[12]

The goal of DP is to reduce dorsal height and convexity without disrupting the anatomically and functional important KA. Although one may risk oversimplification, it is conceptually practical to compare this idea with existing methods of building demolition in architectural engineering. DP can be analogous to the architectural Kajima Cut and Take Down Method used to demolish tall building and prevent noise and dust pollution.

INDICATION

During clinical evaluation, the rhinoplasty surgeon must first decide if DP is a viable option. The question is not just how to remove the hump, but more integral to PR philosophy, how does one keep the dorsum intact? As proposed by Saban,[2] the first step in decision-making and technique selection should be based on nose type and dorsal profile lines (**Table 1**). In brief, four types of noses with corresponding PR and septoplasty technique have been presented. Type 1 PR is full DP with no skin or soft tissue elevation and is best applied to straight noses. Type 2 PR is DP with hump resurfacing allowing for rhinion shift and removal of the bony cap, allowing for better extension at the keystone osteocartilaginous joint. Type 2 PR is recommended for tension noses. We have previously described the management of tension nose in great detail.[13] Type 3 PR described disarticulation techniques (eg, "ballerina maneuver"[14]) to counteract the spring effect and is recommended for humpy kyphotic noses. Finally, Saban recommends structural techniques (or Cottle type procedures for advanced PR surgeons) for difficult noses. Our experience has shown that following this classification approach reduces revisionary rate significantly (**Figs. 2 and 3**).

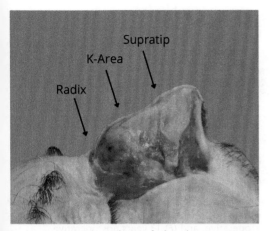

Fig. 1. Segmental analysis of the dorsum. K-Area: keystone area. Cadaveric dissection to demonstrate the above-labeled sections of the dorsum, namely the radix, keystone area, and supratip. Note the difference in soft tissue thickness over the radix compared with the supratip area. The keystone area in the dorsum (aka DKA) denotes the chondro-osseous joint formed by the nasal bones and the upper lateral cartilages.

COMPLICATIONS IN DORSAL PRESERVATION
Functional Concerns

Not every untoward outcome after rhinoplasty requires revisionary surgery. Many of these morbidities resolve with time and conservative management. It is therefore useful to assess these concerns over a time continuum. Although the

Table 1
Basic paradigm for technical recommendation based on nasal morphology

Nose Morphology	Technical recommendation
Straight	Full dorsal preservation
Tension nose deformity	DP + hump resurfacing
Kyphotic/humpy noses	Bony hump resection + KA cartilaginous PD
Twisted and difficult noses	Classical rhinoplasty + mid-vault reconstruction or Cottle's technique

Abbreviations: DP, dorsal preservation; KA, keystone area, PD, push down. (*From* Saban Y, de Salvador S. Guidelines for dorsum preservation in primary rhinoplasty. Facial Plast Surg. 2021;37(1):56.)

focus of this article is evaluation of the long-term results in DP, a brief discussion of early and transient concerns is of value (**Table 2.**)

Early postoperative nasal obstruction is the most common early functional finding. Usually resulting from nasal and turbinate mucosal edema, early nasal obstruction is generally self-resolving within the first 3 months, although intranasal corticosteroids in select cases may hasten the recovery. Although nasal obstruction caused by turbinate hypertrophy in the early postoperative phase may be edematous in nature and transient, persistent turbinate hypertrophy related to bony section or mucosal redundancy may require surgical inferior turbinoplasty to relieve this functional obstruction.

The often transient olfactory disruptions post-rhinoplasty may also be due to internal lining edema in the early postoperative period. Long-lasting anosmia or hyposmia, however, may be related to septal or bony maneuvers that directly or indirectly damage the cribriform area. In our series, four patients complained of long-term anosmia but no clinical or radiographic skull base or cribriform injury was detected.

Persistent nasal obstruction may also be attributed to residual septal deviation, which additionally may cause axis deviation. In these cases, a revisionary surgical septoplasty may likely be required. Given the minimal mucoperichondrial dissection and cartilage harvest in DP with superior strip, revisionary septoplasty is less technically challenging with lesser risk for mucosal perforation and septal instability than in classical septorhinoplasties.

Stenorhinia, or excessively narrow pyriform aperture, has been found in just under 3% of our patients preoperatively. We recommend patients suspected of stenorhinia (clinically or by computed tomography [CT]) be evaluated and counseled regarding the finding, even in the absence of preoperative nasal obstruction as precise preoperative planning and surgical modifications may be needed to prevent postoperative obstructive symptoms. It is important to note that the PDO does not cause pyriform narrowing any more than the classical infracting of the nasal bones.

Esthetic Concerns

As with any esthetic surgery, it is crucial that we have a frank discussion with our patients about their expectations and desired esthetic goals. It is important that the patient is asked to verbalize a hierarchy of their esthetic concerns and expectations, in the order of importance. As surgeons, we

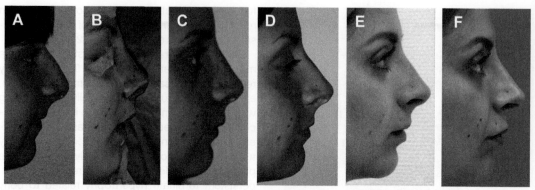

Fig. 2. Chronologic progress profile view of patient undergoing Type 2 dorsal preservation. Note the stability of the dorsal shape over time. (*A*) Preoperative image, (*B*) immediate postoperative result, (*C*) two weeks postoperatively, (*D*) three month postoperative result, (*E*) 8 years postoperative, and (*F*) 13 years postoperative.

must be candid in our review of realistic expectations, healing trajectory and timeline, importance of following postoperative instructions, as well as the possibility of encountering postoperative concerns that may or may not require intervention.

Much of the rhinoplasty final outcome depends on postoperative healing and as such it is crucial for our patients to understand that together with the surgeon they are a team with the common goal of improving their esthetic (and function). In this day and age of social media and unattainable standards of "perfection," it is paramount that our patients are educated to set a realistic goal of substantial "improvement" rather unachievable "perfection." Of course, a psychological analysis of the patient is important to understand motivations and expectations and to rule out concerns such as body dysmorphic disorder before engaging in a surgical intervention.

In similar logic as management of functional concerns, given the healing changes occurring over time, esthetic concerns are also best evaluated across time continuum. In the early stages, periosteal and/or perichondreal fibrotic reactions may create a pseudohump, especially if the

dorsum was accessed for resurfacing. These convexities can be managed by judicious triamcinolone injections. Similarly, fullness in the tip/supratip may be managed by the same in the early postoperative period. Another transient postoperative finding of concern may be related to small areas of cutaneous depression, often along the sidewalls or the radix but may present along the dorsum as well. This minor depression may be ameliorated initially by gentle self-massage and later if required by in-office injection of dissolvable dermal fillers. Other minor irregularities, often caused by bony or cartilaginous spicules may be managed by needle access or gentle rasping under local anesthetic to disrupt the spicule and allow for better contour. Resulting inflammatory reaction may be managed by targeted dilute triamcinolone injections followed-up short-term taping.

Esthetic Concerns Requiring Surgical Intervention: Analysis of our Series

The most important indicators of success in DP are (1) in-depth understanding and candid management of patient expectations, (2) accurate

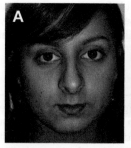 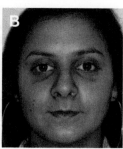 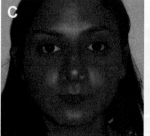 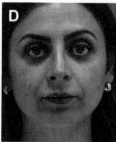

Fig. 3. Chronologic progress frontal view of the same patient shown in Image 2. Note the stability of the dorsal lines over time. (*A*) Preoperative image, (*B*) two weeks postoperative result, (*C*) three months postoperatively, (*D*) three month postoperative result, and (*D*) 13 years postoperative.

Table 2
Transient and permanent functional complications in dorsal preservation

Finding	Early (<3 mo)	Late (more than 3 mo)	Comments
Nasal obstruction	Usually related to mucosal edema. Self-resolving. May consider nasal corticosteroids	Related to residual septal deviation, inferior turbinate hypertrophy and mucosal redundancy.	Nasal valve stenosis or collapse is not a complication normally seen in DP.
Hyposmia/anosmia	Edematous in nature and self-resolving	May be related to obstructive causes or damage to the cribriform/olfactory filaments	In our series, 4 patients developed long-term anosmia. CT did not show skull base injury.
Stenorhinia	Will require surgical intervention if symptomatic	Will require surgical intervention if symptomatic	Although rare, important to consider preoperative CT for surgical planning.

dorsal and nasal analysis, (3) appropriate selection of surgical technique as per guidelines,[2] (4) meticulous surgical execution, and (5) careful postoperative management. Although achieving all esthetic and functional goals in one surgery is the holy grail in rhinoplasty, it is important to educate patients about the possibility of requiring a secondary procedure in cases of complication or dissatisfactory outcomes as even in the best of hands, unexpected healing and fibrosis may result in undesirable results ranging from minor issues to significant complications.

From January 2011 to June 2019, 1210 septorhinoplasties have been performed by the senior author; 672 were primary rhinoplasties done following dorsum preservation procedure using the superior strip PDO. In 272 patients (40.47%), a concomitant Cottle's low strip procedure was performed to correct severe septal deviations. Patient ages ranged from 13 to 71 year old, with 29 as our mean age with a 9 to 1 female-to-male ratio and postoperative follow-up ranging from 3 to 11 years (**Table 3**.)

Technical summary: All cases were performed using the endonasal approach. In Type 1, straight profile noses (n = 188, 28%), no undermining of the skin STE (SSTE) was performed, whereas SSTE undermining was performed in Type 2 (tension noses, n = 121) and in cases of Type 3 kyphotic noses or distorted dorsal esthetic lines (DAL) (n = 128, 37%) to access the dorsum for resurfacing.

Complex dorsal and septal deviation was seen in 235 patients (35%) of which 143 showed straight axis deviation (61%) with 92 showing a C-shape deformity (39%). In these patients, Cottle's low strip procedure concomitant with a high strip (when septum was stable) was performed in an effort to achieve the most optimal profile alignment, which is generally more difficult to obtain in case of low strip as a stand-alone procedure (**Table 4**). In patients with unstable septum, patients underwent structural rhinoplasty, not included in this series.

Analysis of the surgical revisions shows 6.85% global revision rate (46/672). The highest rate of revision was observed in female patients' ages 30 to 39 (21/46%, 46%). Time from surgery to execution of the revision ranged from 6 months to 10 years postoperatively with a mean of 11 months. The case of revision after 10 years was related to the patient's absence as he had moved abroad and was not available for revision at an earlier time. In our series, most of the postoperative issues were successfully managed in office, in the early postoperative period.

The main esthetic or functional concerns in our series are summarized in **Table 5**. In total, 46 of the 672 patients required a surgical revision, constituting a 6.85% revision rate. Our postoperative revision timing ranged from 6 months to 10 years postoperatively, with a mean of 11 months.

Persistent or Recurrence of the Hump

We have previously mentioned the transient causes of hump or pseudohump prominences related to inflammatory or callus formation. However, when a true dorsal convexity either recurs or is noted to be residual due to intraoperative failure of resolving the hump, a revisionary procedure is required. A careful physical examination is paramount to ensure the irregularity is a true dorsal

Table 3
Series demographics

Total number of PDO	672
Date range	2011–2019
Age range	13–71 (mean 29)
Female:male ratio	9:1
Follow-up	3–11 y

Abbreviation: PDO, push down operation.

hump and not a low radix or supratip saddling masquerading as hump.

Intraoperatively, it is important to maintain a gentle hand and strive for minimal dissection and trauma to the tissues as tissue edema, especially in the area of the radix or supratip may camouflage a residual hump which then is seen in the postoperative period once the edema subsides.

One can differentiate between two different biomechanics that may lead to hump persistence or recurrence: (1) framework: cartilage and/or bony structures are involved in the hump persistence and (2) soft tissues are intervening in the shape memory and are responsible of hump recurrence.

If intraoperatively a dorsal hump is noted to be persistent, assuming appropriate patient and technique selection, the surgeon should consider the "problem areas" discussed later in this article

to ensure proper flexion and stretching at the K-Area. In the postoperative period, some additional maneuvers may be required to solve the issue and to keep the patient's trust and confidence.

- *Failure to erase the hump: failure in bony cap removal or in cartilaginous prominence reduction*

Presence of a bony cap over the K-area osteocartilaginous joint may prevent flexion by virtue of the presence of bony thickening over the dorsal K-area. This is often the case in S-shaped nasal bones and requires rasping to remove the bony cap, allowing for flexion at the joint to eliminate dorsal convexity. There are two main goals of this bony resurfacing over the KA: to reduce bony thickness and hump and to produce a rhinion-shift cephalad that will ease further flattening maneuvers. It is for this reason that following technique guidelines set forth is paramount in minimizing complications. In our experience, tension noses or kyphotic noses always require bony cap resurfacing or even resection.

When a bony dorsal convexity is seen in the postoperative period and is persistent beyond the first few weeks, an early revisionary procedure can be performed, within the first 6 months. In our series, we had 21 dorsal hump recurrences or persistences, of which 12 constituted a bony prominence and 9 were cartilaginous. We did not

Table 4
Composition of nasal morphology and techniques used in our series

Nasal Morphology	N	Technique	Comments
Type 1 (straight noses)	188/672 (28%)	Full dorsal preservation, superior strip PDO	
Type 2 (TND)	121/672 (18%)	Superior strip PDO, dorsal resurfacing	
Type 3 (kyphotic noses) or irregular DALs	128/672 (19%)	Superior strip PDO, dorsal resurfacing, lateral disarticulating maneuvers	
Dorsal deviations and difficult noses	235/672 (35%)	Concomitant Cottle's low strip in addition to superior strip and PDO	Straight axis deviation 143/235 (61%) C-shaped septal deformity 92 (39%) Note: Cottle's low strip was only performed in cases with stable septa. If septum was not stable, structural rhinoplasty was used (not included in this series.)

Abbreviations: DAL, dorsal esthetic lines; PDO, push down operation.

Table 5
Postoperative analysis of functional and esthetic results

Postoperative Concern	Number of Patients	Percent of Revisions (x/46)	Percent of Total Patients (x/672)	Time to Revision	Comments
Persistence or recurrence of the bony hump	12	26.1%	1.78%	Between 2–6 mo postoperatively	Simple endonasal rasping sufficient in all bony cases. Sharp shaving of the cartilage in cases of failure of medical therapy.
Persistence or recurrence of cartilaginous hump	9	19.6%	1.33%		
Axis deviations of the dorsum without concomitant nasal obstruction	14	30.4%	2.1%	After 12 mo	
Middle third widening	4	8.7%	0.6%	After 12 mo	
Supratip Saddling	3	6.5%	0.45%	Within first 3 mo	
Bony step offs	2	4.35%	0.3%	Within first 6 mo	
Nasal obstruction (without concomitant axis deviation)	2	4.35%	0.3%	Within first 6 mo	
Anosmia	4	N/A	N/A	Did not require surgical intervention	CT and exam negative for skull base injury
Nostril flaring	1	N/A	N/A	Pt content with outcome; did not require surgical intervention	NB this finding is only noted when tip deprojecting maneuvers have been performed and is not a DP complication per se.

differentiate between recurrence and persistence as such differentiation would not affect the management postoperatively. In one case, revisionary surgery was performed as early as 2 months postoperatively due to psychological reasons. In all bony cases, simple in-office rasping under local anesthesia, with or without mild sedation, satisfactorily resolved the bony convexity. The procedure usually takes less than 10 minutes and does not require significant dissection and tissue manipulation.

Convexity in the cartilaginous portion of the nasal dorsum caudal to the K-area may be related either to true cartilage prominence or to fibrosis in this area. As mentioned, conservative and medical management often improves or resolves most unwanted prominences. In cases of persistent convexity, a careful endonasal shaving by intercartilaginous introduction, the blade of the scalpel under local anesthetic can help achieve resolution of the hump. We had four such cases in our series. In smaller cartilaginous irregularities of the dorsum, transcutaneous shaving with the tip of 18g needle under local anesthesia can be useful (five cases in our series). We generally perform dorsal cartilaginous revisions around 6 months to allow time for medical therapy. In such cases, we have observed fibrocartilaginous production in the high septal area that did not exist preoperatively and could correspond to a healing process of the perichondrium–cartilaginous system similar to a cartilaginous polly beak mechanism. These findings led us to recommend percutaneous injection of triamcinolone in the early postoperative period in the interseptal areas before considering revisionary surgery.

- Coat Hanger Effect

Coat hanger effect refers to the resistance to flattening of the K-area due to the presence of dorsal septal cartilage supporting the convexity above. Residual dorsal septum underneath the K-area may cause a coat hanger effect, thereby resisting flexion at the joint. Intraoperatively, careful examination of the undersurface of the DKA is critical to check some septal remnants underneath the cartilaginous vault. In such cases, complete cleaning of the residual cartilaginous high septum staying remained attached underneath the cartilaginous vault using rongeur forceps; weakening of this subdorsal area is helpful with a few targeted vertical chondrotomies and/or careful slices with a #15 blade to weaken the cartilage in that area.

In the postoperative period, persistent bony-cartilaginous hump appearance may be related to this coat hanger effect and will require further surgical revision including the septal approach and subdorsal cleaning of the cartilaginous remnants.

- The Spring Effect

The spring effect corresponds to the tendency of bony cartilaginous convexity, that is, nasal hump to reappear intraoperatively or postoperatively. The difference with hump persistence is that the convexity fully disappears after surgical manipulations but reappears after a short period of time. Intraoperatively, the spring effect may be related to the failure to release soft tissues. In such cases, the hump may appear softer or even appear fully eliminated but gently reappearing after a very short period of time during the procedure. Therefore, it is crucial that the surgeon addresses all area of resistance be fully released to allow for descent of the bony vault. These include the pyriform ligament and the lateral KA (LKA).[14] In addition, the mucosal and periosteum on the undersurface of the nasal bones may prevent adequate descent. These areas can be gently and safely dissected by use of a small periosteal elevator introduced endonasally.

In cases where the dorsal convexity was completely resolved intraoperative, it is important to remember that the nasal bony pyramid has a tendency to "pop up" during the healing period, resulting in the recurrence of the hump. Thus, it is crucial that the neodorsum is fixed in the proper position until healing takes place. Multiple stabilization techniques have been described including direct and indirect (percutaneous) suturing of the neodorsum to the intact septum. Postoperative splints and taping may also help.

With keeping these principles and concepts in the foreground and with proper execution, remarkable long-term stability is achieved with DP technique (Images 2 and 3.)

Axis Deviations of the Dorsum

Definition

The ideal nasal dorsum runs along a straight perpendicular line dividing the face in two equal vertical halves. Divergence of the nasal dorsum to one side or the other of the midline is considered a lateral deviation of the axis. Lateral deviations of the dorsum after DP may be related to the asymmetric performance or healing of the push down (PDO) Residual septal deviation, especially caudally and dorsally, may also result in axis deviation of the dorsum. Careful performance of PDO, adequate fixation, and proper septoplasty help prevent this untoward complication. If the deviation is related to the asymmetry of nasal bone heights, then asymmetric PDO or unilateral wedge resection (as in LDO) in conjunction with PDO may be indicated in the primary surgery. The Cottle truism "as the septum goes, so goes the nose" was stressed by Gubisch that nasal deviations are always associated or related to septal deformities.

In our series, a total of 14 cases of postoperative axis deviation was noted requiring revisionary surgery (2.1% of all cases.) When axis deviation is noted in the early phase, "digital osteoplasty" may be performed with gentle and steady pressure in office even without local anesthetic. If not possible, the tweak may be performed under anesthesia, and often may not require repeat osteotomy. If the finding is late (even over 3 months) repeat osteotomy has never been mandatory in our experience. Precise clinical and CT-scan evaluation of the high septum is often required to ensure an effective surgical revision. However, in our practice, we could surprisingly perform these office digital osteoplasties even after 2 years post-op; this is probably related to a pseudoarthrosis mechanism in the bony healing process. This office maneuver should be tried before every returning to the operating room.

When a superior strip is performed, the neodorsum may overlap on one side or the other of the intact septum. Intraoperatively, the surgeon must decide laterality as it may have an effect on dorsal esthetics. One can allow the neodorsum to lie to the left or right and evaluate the dorsal axis before fixation. Further, the fixation of the neodorsum to the intact septum should be done with adequate suture tension. If done too loosely, the spring effect will prevail. Done too tightly, the suture may tilt the dorsum to the side of the knot.

If significant, the lateral deviations may be observed in the early postoperative period. However, often this deviation is masked by early edema and becomes visible in a matter of weeks. Conversely, a late deviation secondary to fibrosis may be observed.

Revisionary surgery involving the nasal bones may require repeat osteotomies only followed by fixation of the neodorsum. If the deviation involves the cartilaginous septum, then we must address the septum directly. Although not seen in our series, theoretically in dorsal deviations, placement of asymmetric or bilateral spreader grafts may be required. In these cases, the surgeon should consider a structural or hybrid approach to address the deviation if targeted weakening of the cartilage in areas of deflection does not provide sufficient straightening. Cartilaginous deviations related to C-shaped curvature of the septum may be corrected by incision and overlap of the septum superiorly or inferiorly as recently presented in series by Saman.[15] Furthermore, the swinging door technique may be used to mobilize the septum into a more midline position. Supplemental techniques such as camouflage grafts and clocking sutures can also be of value. In our hands, most revisions were performed at around 1 year to the satisfactory correction of deviation and no further procedure thereafter was needed.

Middle Third Widening

Early postoperative middle third widening could be related to edema and can be managed conservatively with digital massages, taping, possible triamcinolone injections, and the tincture of time. In persistent cases of middle vault fullness, however, surgical revision may be considered. This widening is often noted on the frontal view resulting in a flared nasal shape after PDO. In these patients, the profile contours are satisfactory, contrary to what may be seen in the setting of polly beak deformity.

One cause of middle third widening may be related to excess or overlap of fibrocartilaginous tissue in the scroll area after PDO, a phenomenon we previously have described as the concept of "scroll-winding effect,"[16] whereby scar tissue formation in the proximal scroll area, corresponding to the W-point, or excessive overlap of the caudal ULC scroll at the junction of ULC with LLC, results in tissue excess in the middle third. If medical therapy fails, definitive treatment of this untoward finding is by surgical resection of the excessive tissue.

Alternatively, middle third widening may be attributable to bowing of the ULCs after PDO, thereby widening the arch of the cartilaginous vault in response to PDO. The surgeon must consider preventive maneuvers during the primary DP procedure to account for this bowing if widening of the middle third is not an intended outcome. The widening of the middle third correlates directly with the amount of push down, that is, dorsal height reduction, and logically this effect is exaggerated in patients with cartilaginous noses and short nasal bones. It must be noted that the widening is not always undesired as it can improve the esthetics of a narrow vault and widen the internal valve: an advantage of DP over structural techniques in such cases.

Our case series show a total of four cases of middle third widening requiring surgical intervention (0.6% of all cases). Controlled division of the caudal portion of the ULC from the septum helps prevent cartilaginous vault widening in primary DP procedures. This maneuver effectively moves the W-point cephalically (thus the W-point shift[16]) and increases the length of the W-ASA. In our experience, shorter W-ASA segments are associated with widening. Associated with this W-point shift maneuver is the supplemental partial resection of the ULC scroll which decreases the volume and tension on the ULC/septal junction.

Goksel advocates LKA disarticulation and ULC lateral shift as a mean of not only to control the middle third widening but also to prevent the spring effect.[16] Further, ULC narrowing sutures (horizontal mattress) may help in preventing the widening of (or narrowing the width of) the ULC arch.

During revisionary surgery in cases of middle third widening, the surgeon must debulk the excess scroll volume if indicated in cases attributable to scroll-winding effect. Caudal release of the ULC from the septum with appropriate excision, use of narrowing sutures, and lateral release of the ULC from nasal bones are other tools in our armamentarium to address widening attributable to bowing of the ULCs.

Supratip Saddling

The W-ASA segment functions are a support mechanism for the supratip region. If the superior strip incision is started at the ASA, the descent of the dorsum will drop the W-ASA height, resulting in loss of support in the supratip area. For this reason, we recommend always starting at the W-point to maintain appropriate W-ASA height. Once the dorsum is lowered to appropriate height, W-ASA height can be adjusted by incremental direct excisions of the cartilage thereby managing supratip height. Again, prevention is better than the cure. Should supratip saddling be noted intraoperatively, it can be corrected by solid or diced cartilage grafting.

We had three cases of supratip saddling in our series. Supratip saddling may not be readily identifiable during the immediate or early postoperative period as the structural deficiency may be camouflaged by the swelling in this region. In very minor cases, the saddling may self-resolve with time, probably secondary to deposition of scar tissue in the supratip area. Diagnostically, it is paramount that the surgeon recognizes supratip saddling when present and not confuse it with hump recurrence. Although we have never required it, in the postoperative period, in-office augmentation with hyaluronic acid dermal fillers—or more long-lasting semi-permanent fillers such as polymethylmethacrylate microspheres may be achieved. Permanent augmentation using fat or cartilage may be performed under local anesthesia. Alternatively, the structural deficiency may be addressed by structural grafting.

Bony Steps

Bony steps can be seen in areas of osteotomy, most often in the area of the radix osteotomy but can be seen in the areas of lateral osteotomy (PDO) and less commonly in the area of transverse osteotomy as well. We have two cases of radix bony step off discovered in the postoperative period which was resolved with simple in-office rasping. It is crucial that the surgeon checks these areas of palpable/visible step offs intraoperatively where simple rasping can often improve the contours and avoid revisionary surgery. Rasping or careful infracturing of proud segments may be performed in the postoperative period under local anesthesia or in the operating room. Radix osteotomy location is critical regarding the risk of step deformity. To avoid this issue, the osteotomy must be performed cephalically to the intercanthal line. The direction of the osteotome is important as well. If perpendicular to the sellion, radix can drop; if oblique downward, a hinge is thus created that significantly reduces the risk of dropping. However, if an undesired step occurs, the simplest approach in correcting the issue is to perform another osteotomy through the same percutaneous approach, cutting the bone at a higher level tangential to the glabella, and to drop the bony fragment in the fracture. The same procedure can be easily done percutaneously after to high lateral osteotomies. We refer to these percutaneous osteotomies "rescue percutaneous osteotomies."

REVISIONARY SURGERY AFTER DORSAL PRESERVATION

Preservation *per se* is not able to modify the shape of the bones (weak point) that are strong and rigid. Thus, it is unable to straighten nasal bones and strong or wide cartilages, and consequently bony reshaping or partial resection become inevitable. Conversely, it allows for cartilage remodeling or plication and makes revisions simple (strong points). Therefore, preservation is a perfect procedure for straight noses, cartilaginous noses, nice dorsal lines, and internal nasal valve protection. On the contrary, resection techniques with or without reconstruction allow for removing the deformities (strong point) but weaken the dorsal lines and nasal valve (weak points), thus requiring specific procedures to restructure the areas. This is the rationale for procedures mixing preservation and structure.

DISCUSSION

DP is not appropriate for all nose types and correct patient selection is paramount in preventing complications. However, in discussing long-term results, one can logically deduce that the less the resection and dissection, the less damage to the soft tissues and the less pursuant fibrosis and distortion, all of which make for better long-term results.

It bears reiterating that the most important indicators of success in DP are (1) in-depth understanding and candid management of patient expectations, (2) accurate dorsal and nasal analysis, (3) appropriate selection of surgical technique, (4) meticulous surgical execution, and (5) careful postoperative management.

The dorsal reduction using DP is an effective technique with excellent esthetic outcomes in the long term. It goes without saying that the rhinoplasty surgeon must have deep understanding of nasal anatomy, biodynamics of DP and technical nuances and philosophy of DP for excellent results. When the correct DP technique is applied to the appropriate nose type, the results are astonishingly satisfactory and long-lasting with no patients presenting after 2 years for revisionary surgery in our series. It must be remembered that every nose is different and in considering DP techniques for the inexperienced surgeon, we recommend avoiding the pitfall of forcing indications of DP on all noses. Some noses are simply not optimally addressed with these techniques and require structural rhinoplasty for best results and avoidance of short- and long-term complications.

Therefore, it is critical that the surgeon considers the strengths and weaknesses of various techniques and applies them in such a way that minimizes risks of complications while maximizing benefits to the patient. In DP, bony reshaping may not be as effectively possible as resective techniques. Conversely, PR allows for cartilage modification and contour changes to the dorsum without negatively affecting the internal nasal valves or requiring extensive cartilage grafting which may make revision surgery less complicated.

The first step in decision-making in regard to technique selection should be based on nose type. A practical guideline has been previously published,[2] which should be followed. As with any technique, there will be a learning curve for the surgeon implementing DP into their practice. This discussion will not include technical "errors" but rather is a review of long-term outcomes using the superior strip technique championed by Saban in experienced hands.

Rhinoplasty is as much art as it is science. Although objective measurements of nasal airflow, dorsal height, axis and septal deviation, and more are important, we hold that the most important endpoint is the subject surgeon and patient satisfaction. Our series account of this subjective endpoint indirectly through request or need for revisionary surgery. Additional objective studies are needed to account for objective long-term outcomes in DP.

The most common esthetic complications in DP in our experience were hump recurrence and lateral deviations of the dorsum. A discussion of these complications, as well as other less commonly seen complications in DP, has been provided. None of our cases required complex revisions or requiring rib grafting. In our analysis of long-term results in patients who have undergone superior strip DP, a striking finding is the absence of classic complications such as open roof deformity, inverted V deformity, polly beak deformity, and nasal valve stenosis, all of which usually require complex revisionary surgery. In our experience, DP rhinoplasty results in high long-term patient and surgeon satisfaction with lower revision rates compared with classical rhinoplasty. Further, the abundance of available septal cartilage in DP makes revisionary surgery simpler and safer than in structural rhinoplasty.

CLINICS CARE POINTS

- The renewed interest in dorsal preservation techniques in recent years has resulted in some lack of consensus on terminology, indications, classifications, and techniques among rhinoplasty surgeons.

- We present long-term data on complications and follow-up after dorsal preservation rhinoplasty.

- Dorsal preservation is not appropriate for all nose types, and correct patient selection is paramount in preventing complications.

- Many of the untoward outcomes following dorsal preservation technique resolve with conservative management and watchful waiting.

- Complications resulting from dorsal preservation rhinoplasty generally require a less involved and technically simpler revisionary procedure, often not requiring additional cartilage grafting, contrary to most complications after structural rhinoplasty techniques.

- Outcomes after dorsal preservation rhinoplasty are very stable with high satisfaction rates for the patient and the surgeon.

DISCLOSURE

The authors have no commercial or financial conflicts of interest or any funding for the production of this article.

REFERENCES

1. Saban Y, Daniel RK, Polselli R, et al. Dorsal preservation: the push down technique reassessed. Aesthet Surg J 2018;38(2):117–31.

2. Saban Y, de Salvador S. Guidelines for dorsum preservation in primary rhinoplasty. Facial Plast Surg 2021;37(1):53–64.

3. Gonçalves Ferreira M, Toriumi DM. A practical classification system for dorsal preservation rhinoplasty techniques. Facial Plast Surg Aesthet Med 2021; 23(3):153–5.

4. Goodale JL. A new method for the operative correction of exaggerated roman nose. Boston Med Surg J 1899;140:112.

5. Lothrop OA. An operation for correcting the aquiline nasal deformity; the use of new instrument; report of a case. Boston Med Surg J 1914;170:835–7.

6. Sebileau P, Dufourmentel L. Surgical correction of congenital and acquired deformities of the nasal pyramid. Paris: Arnette; 1926, p. 104-105. (In French)

7. Maurel G. Chirurgie maxilla-faciale. Paris: Le François; 1940. p. 1127–33.

8. Cottle MH, Loring RM. Corrective surgery of the external nasal pyramid and the nasal septum for restoration of normal physiology. Ill Med J 1946;90: 119–35.

9. Gola R, Nerini A, Laurent-Fyon C, et al. Conservative rhinoplasty of the nasal canopy. Ann Chir Plast Esthet 1989;34(6):465–75.

10. Cottle MH. Nasal roof repair and hump removal. AMA Arch Otolaryngol 1954;60(4):408–14.

11. Palhazi P, Daniel RK, Kosins AM. The osseocartilaginous vault of the nose: anatomy and surgical observations. Aesthet Surg J 2015;35(3):242–51.

12. Saban Y, Andretto Amodeo C, Hammou JC, et al. An anatomical study of the nasal superficial musculoaponeurotic system: surgical applications in rhinoplasty. Arch Facial Plast Surg 2008;10(2):109–15.

13. Saban Y, Saman M. Tension nose deformity. Mediterranean rhinoplasty. SPRINGER; 2022.

14. Goksel A, Saban Y. Open Piezo Preservation Rhinoplasty: A Case Report of the New Rhinoplasty Approach. Facial Plast Surg 2019;35(1):113–8. https://doi.org/10.1055/s-0039-1678578.

15. Saman M. Preservation Rhinoplasty for Beginners. Oral presentation at: Montpellier Rhinoplasty Annual Meeting. May 12-14, 2022.

16. Saban Y, De Salvador S, Polselli R. Revisions following dorsal preservation rhinoplasties. In: Daniel RK, Palhazi P, Saban Y, et al, editors. Preservation rhinoplasty. 3rd edn. Istanbul: Septum; 2020. p. 404–29.

My Approach to Preservation Rhinoplasty

Barış Çakır[a],*, Bülent Genç, MD[b], Valerio Finocchi, MD[c], Sebastian Haack, MD[d]

KEYWORDS

- Preservation rhinoplasty • Dorsal preservation • Ligament preservation • High strip • Low strip
- Endonasal rhinoplasty

KEY POINTS

- Subperichondrial dissection is important to allow proper skin redraping and to prevent scar contracture.
- Preservation of Pitanguy's and scroll ligaments is critical to tip support.
- Preservation of the lateral crus and scroll ligament is critical to avoiding alar retraction.
- The alar rim flap helps to avoid deformities of the alar margin.

The "preservation rhinoplasty" term was coined in 2018 by Rollin K. Daniel's article "The Preservation Rhinoplasty: A New Rhinoplasty Revolution."[1] After consulting with Daniel, we named our meeting in Istanbul, December 2018 as the "Preservation Rhinoplasty Meeting." The First Edition of the Preservation Rhinoplasty Book went on sale on the second day of the meeting. The second and third editions have subsequently been published.[2–4] Thanks to Rollin K. Daniel, some techniques that were described many years ago but forgotten have become popular again. As of July 2022, there are 81 articles about preservation rhinoplasty in the PubMed search engine.

Daniel sums up his preservation rhinoplasty article this way: "We must fundamentally change how we perform rhinoplasty surgery which leads to the next revolution—the preservation rhinoplasty. The fundamental goal is to replace resection with preservation, excision with manipulation, and secondary rib reconstruction with minimal revisions." He also points out suture tip-plasty with minimal resection, lateral crural tensioning with lateral crural steal, minimal excision from the lateral crus, dorsal preservation, subperichondrial dissection, preservation of the Pitanguy and scroll ligaments.[5–13]

I started rhinoplasty surgery in 2004 with the open structure technique. I switched to closed rhinoplasty in 2008. In 2009, I started to protect the Pitanguy and scroll ligaments.[9] I started using the auto-rim flap technique in 2013.[14] I have been using dorsal preservation techniques since 2016. In 2019, I began applying lateral crural preservation techniques.

INCISIONS

The main reason why I prefer the closed technique is to protect the ligaments rather than refraining from the transcolumellar incision. The open rhinoplasty incision does not give me an extra field of view as I perform the surgery while preserving the Pitanguy ligament. Because the columellar system is intact, tip edema resorbs more quickly. To increase the field of view in closed surgery, I lengthen the incision up to the footplates in the medial crura and 1.5 to 2 cm laterally after the turning point in the lateral crura (**Fig. 1**). As I usually operate on big noses, I use bilateral low septal incisions. With the low septal incision, I get a very good field of view in the septum. In 80% to 90% of the cases, I remove the mucosa bilaterally. In this way, I can shorten the nose better and rarely see membranous mucosal thickening. I have not used an intercartilaginous incision in the past 5 years. I reach the ULC and bone through the lateral crura and the lateral osteotomy area by

[a] Teşvikiye Cd., No:3A Güneş Apt. K:1, 34365 Nişantaşı, Şişli, İstanbul, Turkey; [b] Private Practice, Caddebostan Mah Çam Fıstığı Sok No:1 A Blok D:3 34728 Kadıköy, Istanbul, Turkey; [c] Private Practice, Via Isonzo, 32, 00198 Roma RM, Italy; [d] Private Practice, Böheimstraße 37, 70199 Stuttgart, Germany
* Corresponding author.
E-mail address: op.dr.bariscakir@gmail.com

Facial Plast Surg Clin N Am 31 (2023) 25–43
https://doi.org/10.1016/j.fsc.2022.08.014
1064-7406/23/© 2022 Elsevier Inc. All rights reserved.

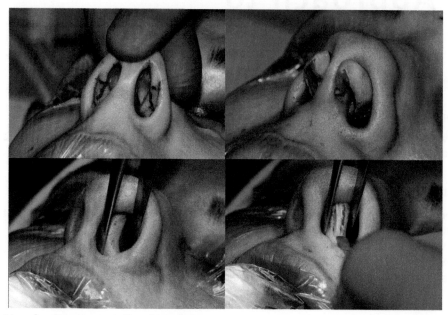

Fig. 1. Incisions for closed preservation rhinoplasty.

dissecting the pyriform ligament from the skin. Wide dissection increases edema but on the other hand increases redrape and decreases bruising.

PRESERVATION OF THE SOFT TISSUE ENVELOPE

The dissection may be subareolar (just over the perichondrium) (Neves C, personal communication, Nice 2021) or subperichondrial at the tip of the nose. I always prefer subperichondrial dissection on the dorsum of the nose. I prefer subareolar dissection in overly bulbous and thick-skinned noses with weak lower lateral cartilages (LLC). Redrape is more prominent after subareolar dissection. It is not easy to shape the cartilages with stitches when the perichondrium is not left on weak cartilages. I prefer subperichondrial dissection in patients with strong LLCs and thin skin. I performed subperichondrial dissection and ligament preservation and observed my long follow-up results. Decrease in the mobility of the nasal skin and appearance of soft tissue atrophy are minimal. You can see 9 year postop of a thin skin patient (Figs. 2–7).

Fibrosis is minimal after subperichondrial dissection. Soft tissue damage is less due to the healing and camouflage effects of the perichondrium. Tissue injury by the pressure of retractors on fat and muscle is also reduced. Soft tissue atrophy and skeletonization are very rare. Preservation of the Pitanguy and scroll ligaments minimizes the loss of definition in the nasal tip whereby subareolar dissection is preferred.

I always do subperichondrial dissection in the dorsum because I can extend the dissection sideways for redrape. The K point, which is whereby most of the irregularity occurs is also where the dorsal perichondrium is the thickest. Subperichondrial dissection provides great camouflage for the dorsum. The biggest advantage of dorsal subperichondrial dissection is the reconstruction of the scroll region. I suture the caudal border of the ULC perichondrium back to the caudal border of the ULC at the end of the surgery (Fig. 8). In this way, I can achieve a reduction in the soft tissue that parallels that of the dorsal cartilage roof. Since no dead space is left, the deprojection of the skeleton is largely reflected on the skin. My rate of steroid injection for supratip deformity is less than 1% in primary rhinoplasty with Pitanguy repair and scroll reinsertion.

Projection loss is reduced to a minimum with the membranous tongue-in-groove technique (Fig. 9). It should be noted that with the ligament-sparing approach, the form you see in the surgery is mostly permanent. Overcorrection should be avoided at the supratip break point and in projection and rotation. But in patients with very thick skin, 3% to 5% overcorrection is advisable.

PITANGUY PRESERVATION

The Pitanguy ligament is formed by the supratip thickening of the nasal SMAS. It passes between the domes and anterior nasal spine (ANS) and adheres to the medial crura. Due to its thickness, it acts as a cushion between the domes and ANS,

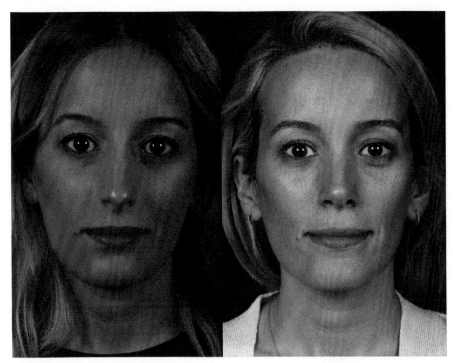

Fig. 2. 9 years postop of a thin skin patient.

pushing the domes forward. It makes a great contribution to the projection and rotation of the nasal tip as it adheres to the medial crura. Preservation of the Pitanguy and scroll system

significantly reduces the amount of graft required for projection and rotation. While it is necessary to cut the Pitanguy ligament in primary augmentation patients, preservation of the Pitanguy

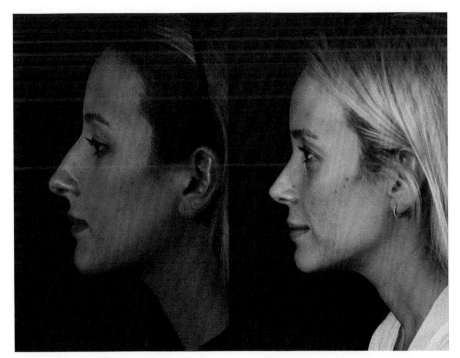

Fig. 3. 9 years postop of a thin skin patient.

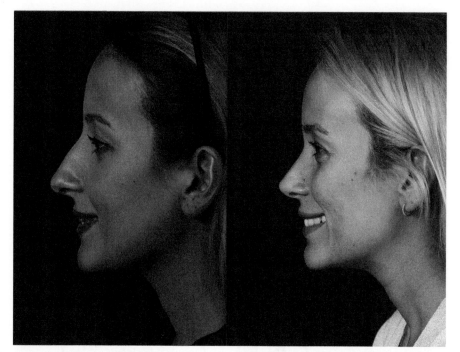

Fig. 4. 9 years postop of a thin skin patient.

ligament in primary reduction patients minimizes the loss of definition.

The Pitanguy ligament determines the distance between the supratip and columellar break point. The middle crura and domes remain above this level and the Pitanguy ligament forms a compartment for the lobule. Therefore, there is an important relationship between the length of

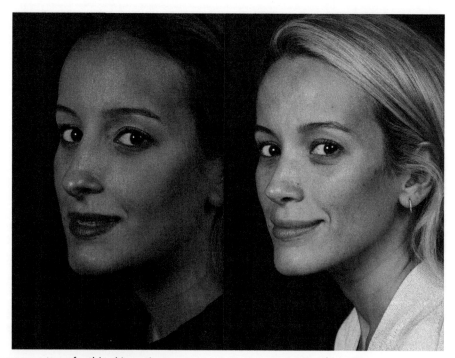

Fig. 5. 9 years postop of a thin skin patient.

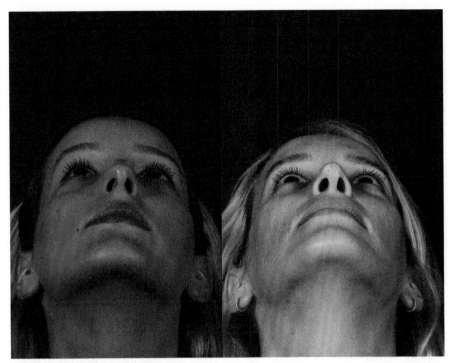

Fig. 6. 9 years postop of a thin skin patient.

the Pitanguy ligament and projection of the lobule. In patients with short lobules, it is necessary to increase the volume of the lobule compartment by increasing the dissection between the deep and superficial Pitanguy ligaments. The ligament compartment, which is slightly smaller than the cartilage skeleton that forms the lobule, provides us with definition.

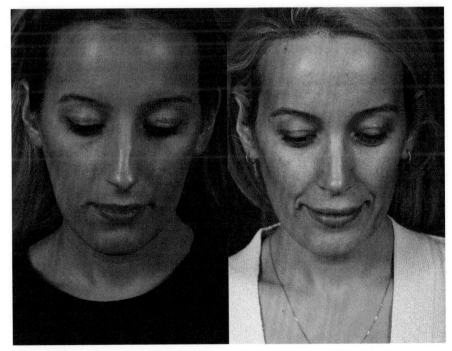

Fig. 7. 9 years postop of a thin skin patient.

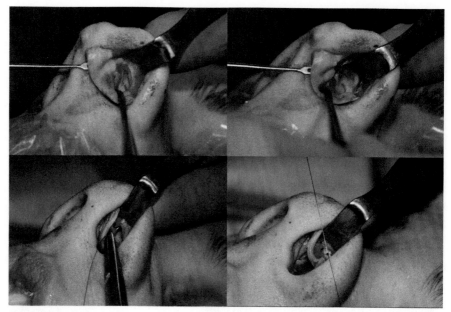

Fig. 8. Scroll ligament repair.

The ideal supratip break point is halfway between the tip and K point. The dissection between the superficial and deep Pitanguy ligaments is conducted up to the planned supratip break point. If there is over-definition at the supratip break point at the end of the tip surgery, the amount of dissection is gradually increased.

Thus, the supratip break point is formed with the original anatomic structure and redrape is kept under control (**Figs. 10** and **11**).

Why does supratip deformity not occur in patients who undergo ligament preservation? The most appropriate explanations that come to mind would be as follows:

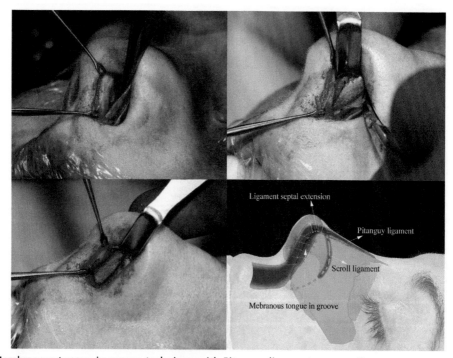

Fig. 9. Membranous tongue-in-groove technique with Pitanguy ligament preservation.

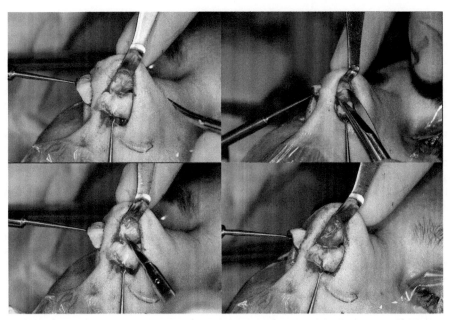

Fig. 10. Pitanguy preservation and setting the tip definition and supratip break point with Pitanguy window dissection amount.

1. The transversalis muscle, one of the largest muscles of the nasal SMAS, wraps the cartilaginous roof like a curtain. The muscle dissected from the floor during a rhinoplasty surgery, collects the soft tissues in the midline and creates a supratip deformity after the muscle starts functioning. As the transversalis muscle is reinserted into the scroll region with the repair of

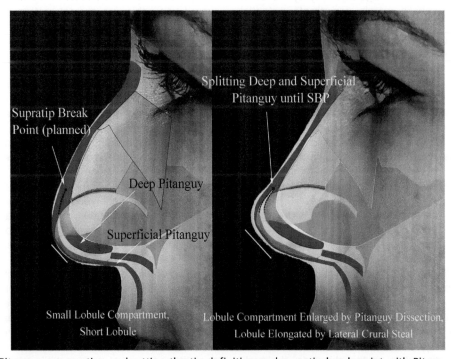

Fig. 11. Pitanguy preservation and setting the tip definition and supratip break point with Pitanguy window dissection amount.

the scroll region and Pitanguy ligament, the negative effect of the muscle on redraping is prevented and internal valve collapse can be minimized by connecting the muscle to the functional internal valve region.

2. The thick supratip skin with its stronger memory may prevent reduction in the supratip skin. Maintaining the connection between the skin and skeleton through the SMAS can counteract the skin's memory. We can somehow think of this as supratip internal taping or quilting sutures. Thus, we can keep the lateral spread of the supratip skin under control in the long term.

LATERAL CRURAL PRESERVATION

In order for the rhinoplasty result to remain stable, I think the width and length of the lateral crura (LC) should be adjusted exactly to the planned nose.

Wide LC: The LC supports the alar rims by taking support from the upper lateral cartilage (ULC). Creating a potential gap between the ULC and LC poses a risk of alar retraction. For this reason, the LC-ULC end-to-end contact at the end of the surgery is important. Even if the LC is wide enough, alar retraction can still occur if it slides over the ULC. Repairing the vertical scroll ligament prevents the LC from sliding onto the ULC (see **Fig. 8**). Treating very large LCs only by resection from the cephalic margin can create potential spaces in the scroll region. Therefore, using a rim flap in patients with caudal excess of the LC reduces the necessary amount of cephalic resection.[14] After I started using the rim flap technique, my alar retraction problems were minimized. In the sliding alar cartilage (SAC) technique, one of the LC preservation techniques, Özmen uses the cephalic excess to strengthen the LC instead of removing it. Since the horizontal scroll ligament is preserved, the LC-ULC relationship becomes more stable. On the other hand, the LC pinching effect of the dome stitches decreases. Flattening to some degree in the LC is also achieved. I think the flattening effect is due to the dissection of the LC from the mucosa. Therefore, I started dissecting the LC subperichondrially from the mucosa and I achieved a more pronounced flattening of the LC. In extremely convex LCs, turn-under or turn-over flaps may be preferred, but to say the least, subperichondrial dissection and SAC flap usually meet my needs. Dr. Shah Nazari says that if subperichondrial dissection is performed on the mucosa side and subSMAS dissection on the skin side, the perichondrium creates a corrective force on the LC

(personal communication June 2022, Istanbul). Subperichondrial dissection on the mucosal side of LC is not easy. To facilitate dissection, I cut 70% to 80% of the SAC flap with a scalpel at an angle of 30 to 40°. After the remaining part of the cartilage is broken with an elevator, the subperichondrial plane can be easily entered. In this plane, the elevator moves very easily. The mucosa does not become overly loose. The most suitable elevator in this region can be the Daniel-Cakir Elevator (Medicon ®) or a very thin semisharp elevator. One or 2 mm chisel can also be used. Note that to perform a lateral steal, it is necessary to cut the tip of the SAC flap (**Fig. 12**).

Long LC: The length of the LC should be equal to the distance between the tip of the nose and lateral supra alar groove (**Fig. 13**). LC should be shortened in noses whereby rotation and deprojection are performed. LC that is overly weakened and left long usually results in a pinch nose. A long LC either collapses inward at its weakest part or causes loss of rotation or lateral bulbosity. I prefer LC steal technique to shorten long LC (**Fig. 14**). I can both do LC tensioning without disturbing the LC continuity and increase lobule projection in patients with short lobules.[12,15] Since I use LC steal with Pitanguy preservation, my incidence of onlay tip grafts in primary reduction rhinoplasty does not exceed 5%. For the LC steal, I combine the cephalic dome and oblique transdomal sutures. In this way, I can achieve a correct resting angle and a natural tip.

DORSAL PRESERVATION

I learned the dorsal preservation technique from Yves Saban in Budapest in 2016. Half of my rhinoplasty surgery has changed thanks to Yves Saban. Although I had problems in the learning process, so far I have achieved my most beautiful nasal dorsums with this technique and I have started to correct crooked noses much better.

Dorsal preservation can be classified according to the structures preserved and the surgery in the septum. The classification can be made as low, intermediate, or superior strip in the septum and cartilage only or osseocartilaginous preservation in the dorsum.

I mostly prefer the low septal strip technique in the septum because I observe deviations at the base of the septum in most of my patients. The low septal strip technique allows us to easily correct the curvatures of the ethmoid bone in crooked noses, and the rotation movement of the septum straightens the nasal dorsum while raising the tip of the nose like a seesaw.

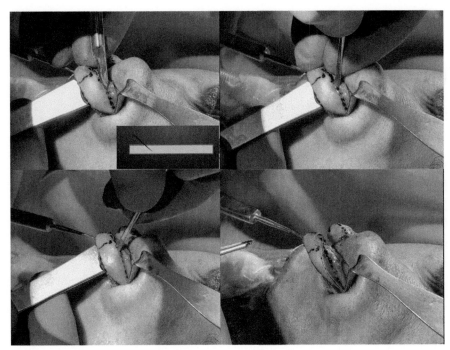

Fig. 12. SAC flap with subperichondrial dissection.

SEPTOPLASTY

I reach the septum with a low septal incision. I remove the low septal strip with a flat lateral osteotome (Fanous-Gubisch lateral osteotome ®); the width of the strip is 1 mm at the anterior maxillary spine and 3 to 4 mm near the vomer bone. With a Cottle elevator, I start the vertical incision whereby the dorsum is the highest. I reach the perpendicular plate of ethmoid (PPE) with an oblique incision

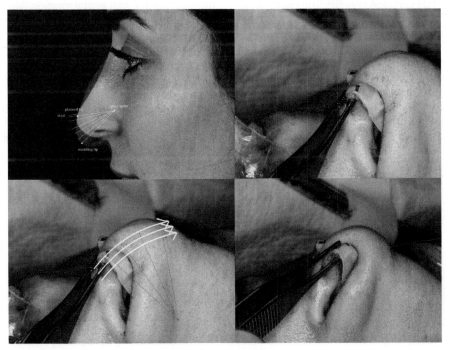

Fig. 13. Treating the long lateral crura with lateral crura steal.

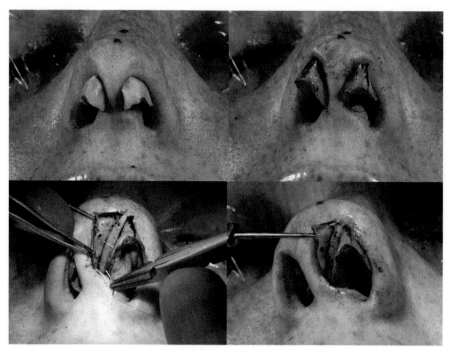

Fig. 14. A summary of tip surgery including lateral crura steal.

and completely separate the septum from the bone. I remove a cartilage triangle from under the bony roof with a 2 mm punch (Weil-Blakesley thru-cutting forceps). At this point, I decide which technique I will prefer on the dorsum. If I need to remove more than 3 mm of bone until the radix osteotomy, I do cartilage only DP. The relationship between the amount of resection and radix osteotomy can be easily measured with the legs of bayonet forceps (Sercan Bayonet Test) (**Fig. 15**). Osseocartilaginous DP can be performed with great safety in cartilage-dominant septums. I rotate the septum as needed and fix it to the anterior maxillary spine with a 4/0 round needle PDS. Passing through the septum 2 to 3 times in the form of a horizontal mattress suture, as suggested

by Carlos Neves, provides a very safe fixation (personal communication, Nice 2021). Resection from the posterior of the septum provides reduction at the K point and anterior resection results in reduction at the supratip area. The posterior septal angle acts as a septal extension flap as it moves caudally with septal rotation. Membranous tongue-in-groove combined with Pitanguy ligament preservation is usually sufficient for rotation and projection control in Caucasian noses.

DORSUM

Osseocartilaginous DP may be preferred in patients whereby both the bony and cartilaginous dorsums are relatively flat and beautiful and the

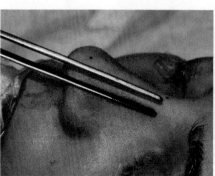
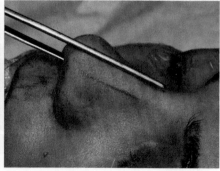

Fig. 15. The relationship between the amount of resection and radix osteotomy can be easily measured with the legs of a bayonet forceps (Sercan Bayonet Test).

PPE is short. I don't dissect the bony dorsum if it is beautiful and delicate enough so that even a rasping is unnecessary (Finocchi, SPQR2). If an intervention on the bone is needed, I reach the area with a tunnel or very wide dissection. I shape the dorsum and do osseocartilaginous DP (Finocchi, SPQR1).[16] If the bony dorsum does not have a good shape or is excessively convex, I only preserve the dorsal cartilage and apply classical resection to the bony dorsum. I close the open bony roof with classical osteotomies.[17] I think this is the most appropriate technique to start dorsal preservation.

Osseocartilaginous DP: If a lateral ostectomy is performed for dorsal reduction, it is called letdown, and if an osteotomy is performed, it is called pushdown. I've tried both, but in recent years I prefer letdown. I try to avoid bony overlap. I have encountered problems such as breathing problems or narrow nasal base in patients with narrow pyriform apertures. In patients with limited lateral dissection, over-defined lateral aesthetic lines may occur due to the periosteum of the bone that slides in. Therefore, I prefer wide dissection from the maxillary groove to the nasal bone suture line. I dissect the pyriform ligament from the skin, exposing the entire caudal edge of the maxillary and nasal bones. I dissect the inside of the bone to be removed with lateral ostectomy for 2.5 to 3 cm in the shape of a banana.

With sharp dissection, I dissect the ULC 3 to 6 mm from the bone subperiosteally. I do not dissect toward the inner part of the nasal passage to stabilize the bone after mobilization. I do the lateral ostectomy in the shape of a banana (banana ostectomy, Sebastian Haack, COVID quarantine Zoom webinars). It is necessary to create a gap in the transverse osteotomy line so that the bone can rotate with the radix as the pivot point instead of detaching from the radix. I make multiple osteotomies with a 1 mm chisel on the stalk end of the banana shape. I remove the Webster triangle with a rongeur. At the level of the nasal bone suture line, I combine the lateral and transverse osteotomies. With a lateral osteotome, I cut along the anterior edge of the banana shape and proceed up to the radix (**Fig. 16**). I place a 1 mm chisel under the radix under direct vision. I make an oblique cut, holding the chisel near the tip of the chin. It is possible to easily feel the tip of the chisel on the radix with the fingertip (**Fig. 17**). Inside out osteotomy makes more sense to me as I do not apply a posterior force to the bone. Another advantage is that I do not need to make an additional incision for the radix osteotomy. The osteotomies so far are usually sufficient for the initial mobilization. To avoid fracture in the midline of the bone, I grasp the nose with 2 fingers as close to the dorsum of the nose as possible and mobilize the dorsum with sideways movements to the right and left. If gentle force is not enough for mobilization, I recheck the osteotomies. At this stage, when looking at the lateral osteotomy site, the areas whereby the bones overlap can be easily seen. As you perform a lateral osteotomy for a 2 mm segment at a time, the osteotome mobilizes bone fragments to follow the shape of the banana. I continue shaving osteotomies until the overlap disappears. I try to create a gap of 1 to 3 mm width. If the bone removal is not treated aggressively, hump recurrence occurs. I have had no problems with removing bone extensively because the periosteum treats this area very well. I examine the cartilage contacts by simulating septal rotation and I usually remove additional low septal strips. I make resections with an Ayhan PPE punch (Medisoft ®, Ankara) without any rotational movements from the areas whereby the septum and PPE overlap. After I started completely separating the septum from the maxilla and ethmoid bone and removing the high bony deviations, crooked noses are no longer my fearful dreams. By releasing all points that cause septal curvature, a kind of intracorporeal septoplasty is performed. You can see 1-year postoperative results of a patient with osseocartilaginous DP (**Figs. 18–22**).

Cartilage only DP: In this technique, the dorsal cartilage is preserved and a classical resection of the bony roof is performed. The entire bony dorsum, the ULC, and the pyriform ligament are dissected in the subperiosteal-subperichondrial plane. It is necessary to create a space whereby the ULC will go laterally. The ULC, including the pyriform ligament, is dissected from the bone subperiosteally as needed. I take great care to protect the internal and external periosteum of the bony cap. When 2 layers of periosteum are protected at the K point, they heal by thickening. This greatly reduces the irregularities at the K point and the need for camouflage. I have seen bony humps form in patients whereby I had placed bone shavings to treat minimal irregularities. If there is a significant depression on the dorsum, I place bone paste produced by a bone rasp without overcorrection.[18]

I rasp the bone polygon with a Cakir bone rasp (Medisoft ®, Ankara) until it is as thin as a bony membrane so that it fits the form of the bony roof. I press the dorsal bony roof with an elevator and mobilize it together with the ULC. The membranous bony cap, which remains above the ULC, creates an anatomic form when the roof is closed. After the cartilage roof has come

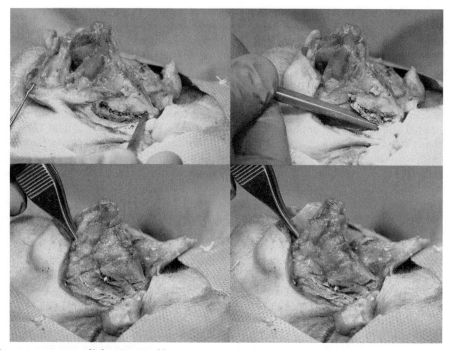

Fig. 16. Banana ostectomy (Sebastian Hack).

down to the appropriate level, I perform a classical resection of the bony roof with bone rongeurs, bone scissors, or chisels. After obtaining the open bony roof at an appropriate height, I thin out the bone edges with the help of a rasp. The fact that the height of the bone flaps are 1 to 2 mm lower at the cartilage level, especially at the K point, creates a more anatomic form. The next step is to close the bony roof in a controlled manner. To make a proper osteotomy, I thin out the lateral osteotomy lines with a Taştan ostectomy rasp (Medisoft ®, Ankara). I also thin out the bone convexities with a bone

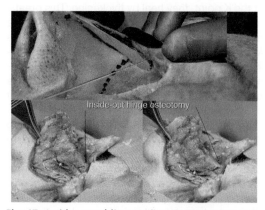

Fig. 17. Inside–out oblique radix osteotomy to create a hinge.

rasp. With a 1 mm chisel, I make external osteotomies in a straight line starting from the open roof to the superior medial canthus. I have difficulty closing the open roof with medial oblique osteotomies from the inside. In my hands, closing the bone roof is easier with external osteotomies made at right angles to the bone. I dissect a tunnel of 2 mm width and 2 cm length under the inner periosteum of the lateral osteotomy line. I start the lateral osteotomy 3 to 4 mm superior to the Webster triangle. I continue the osteotomy until the bone is mobilized. Protecting the inner periosteum by creating a tunnel helps a lot in keeping the bones stable.

If the dorsal cartilage is large, it can be shaped with oblique partial incisions and resection after the mucosa is infiltrated. Below you can find the 2.5-year-postop result of a patient who underwent cartilage-only DP (**Figs. 23–29**).

Low Septal Strip - Robotti: Robotti preserves the dorsal Y cartilage with a high septal strip.[19] I used this technique with a low septal strip in 15 patients. I prefer it for very large noses and patients with very wide and high ULCs. I separate the ULC from the dorsal Y cartilage by dissecting the mucosa subperichondrial. I dissect the septum unilaterally and lower the dorsal Y cartilage. Resections need to be conducted very carefully, because, in this technique, the septum descends very easily as it is only attached to the mucosa. If

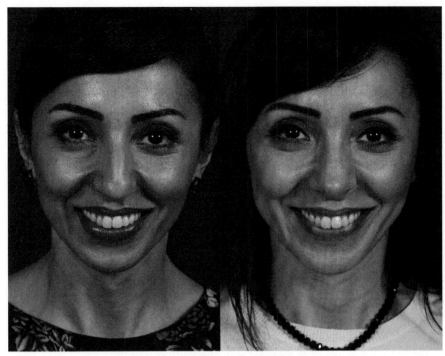

Fig. 18. One-year postoperative results of a patient with osseocartilaginous DP.

the dorsal Y is wide, it is narrowed. The ULC and the bony roof are resected conventionally. The open roof is closed with osteotomies. Usually, there is no need to suture the ULC to the dorsal Y cartilage. Protecting the mucosa especially close to the Y part of the septum is very important for stabilization. I fix the septum loosely to the spine, either without rotation or with minimal

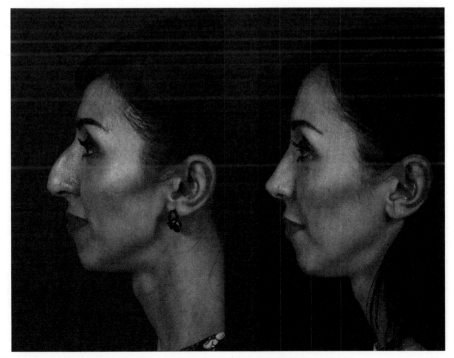

Fig. 19. One-year postoperative results of a patient with osseocartilaginous DP.

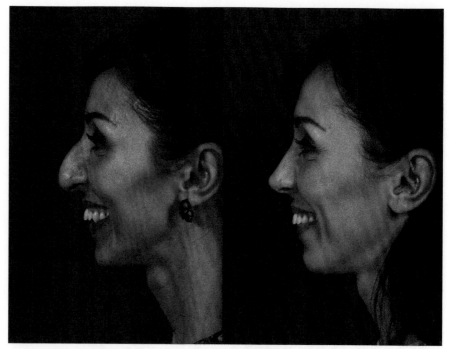

Fig. 20. One-year postoperative results of a patient with osseocartilaginous DP.

rotation. In this technique, the ULC is not dissected from the bone; large amounts of resection are possible and moreover, a fusiform shape of the dorsum can be obtained without dorsal reconstruction.

DRAINS

Wide dissection may reduce bruising to a great extent but may increase edema. For this reason, it is necessary to prevent blood accumulation in

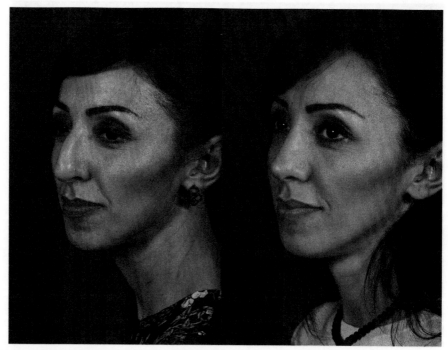

Fig. 21. One-year postoperative results of a patient with osseocartilaginous DP.

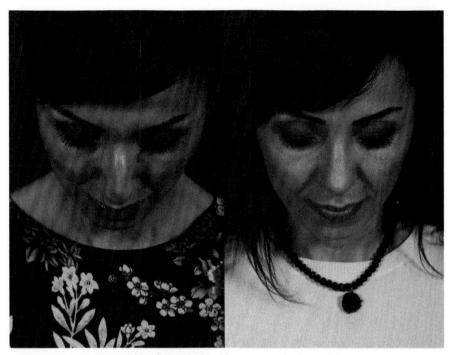

Fig. 22. One-year postoperative results of a patient with osseocartilaginous DP.

the subperiosteal plane for the first 2 to 3 days. I definitely recommend putting a gray iv-catheter into the pocket. I remove the needle and cut off the excess. I lift a proximally based flap of plastic leaving the 5 mm distal end of the catheter uncut. In this way, drainage is facilitated and the plastic flap prevents the drain from moving inside (**Fig. 30**). I enter the lateral

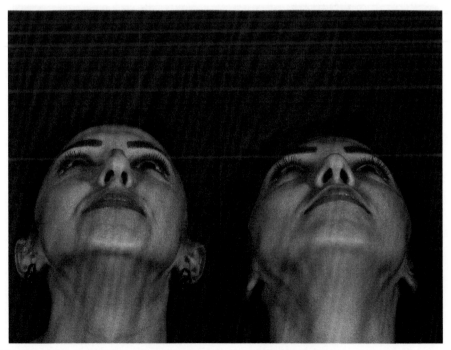

Fig. 23. 2.5-year-postop result of a patient who underwent cartilage-only DP.

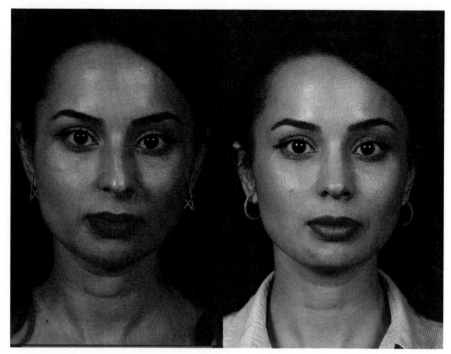

Fig. 24. 2.5-year-postop result of a patient who underwent cartilage-only DP.

osteotomy or ostectomy pouch as if it were vascular access, I keep the Doyle splints for 5 days and external splints for 10 to 12 days. Although I start using cold compresses on the 2nd day, I do not see significant bruising in 90% of my cases. If a large subperichondrial dissection is made in the LC, I recommend a nostril retainer for a month or 2.

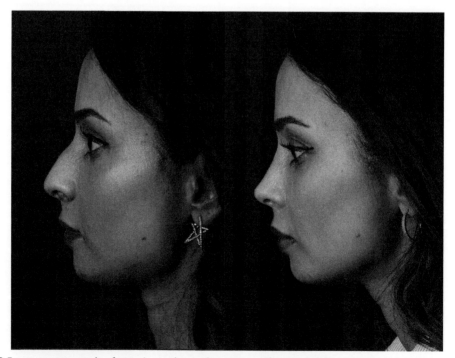

Fig. 25. 2.5-year-postop result of a patient who underwent cartilage-only DP.

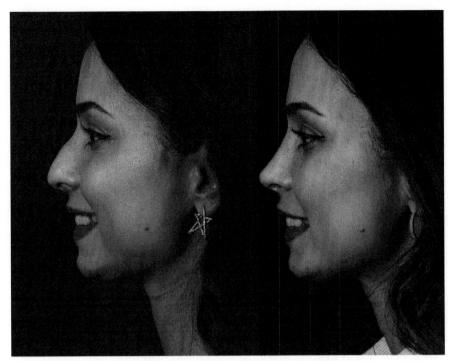

Fig. 26. 2.5-year-postop result of a patient who underwent cartilage-only DP.

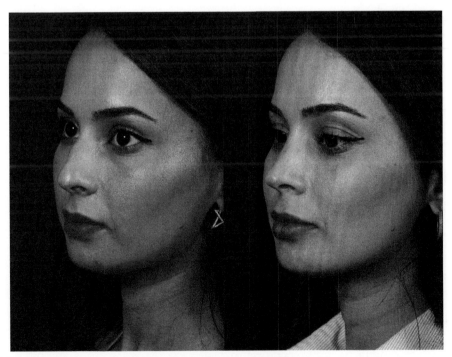

Fig. 27. 2.5-year-postop result of a patient who underwent cartilage-only DP.

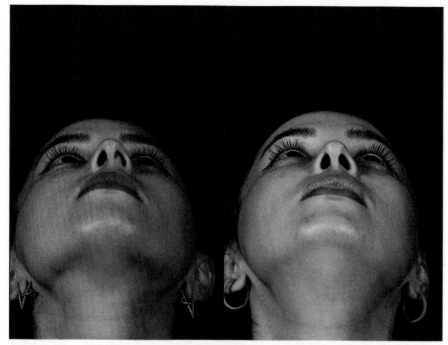

Fig. 28. 2.5-year-postop result of a patient who underwent cartilage-only DP.

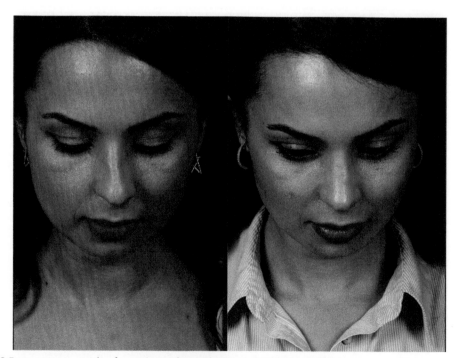

Fig. 29. 2.5-year-postop result of a patient who underwent cartilage-only DP.

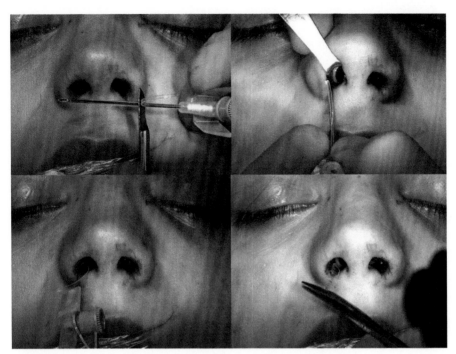

Fig. 30. Placing drains to lateral osteotomy sites to decrease edema and bruising.

For more detailed reading, the 2nd Edition of the Aesthetic Septorhinoplasty Book (Çakır, B., Springer, 2021) can be viewed (18).

REFERENCES

1. Daniel RK. The Preservation Rhinoplasty: A New Rhinoplasty Revolution. Aesthet Surg J 2018 Feb 17; 38(2):228–9.
2. Cakir B, Saban Y, Daniel RK, et al. Preservation rhinoplasty. Istanbul: Septum Publications; 2018.
3. Daniel RK, Palhazi P, Saban Y, et al. Preservation rhinoplasty. Istanbul: Septum Publications; 2020.
4. Saban Y, Cakir B, Daniel RK, et al. Preservation rhinoplasty. Istanbul: Septum Publications; 2019.
5. Daniel RK, Palhazi P. The nasal ligaments and tip in rhinoplasty: an anatomical study. Aesthet Surg J 2018;38(4):357–68.
6. Palhazi P, Daniel RK, Kosins AM. The osseocartilaginous vault of the nose: anatomy and surgical observations. Aesthet Surg J 2015;35(3):242–51.
7. Saban Y, Polselli R. Atlas d'Anatomie Chrirurgicale de la Face et du Cou. Florence, Italy: SEE Editrice; 2009.
8. Cakir, B. (2016) Aesthetic Septorhinoplasty. Springer.
9. Cakir B, Oreroglu AR, Dogan T, et al. A complete subperichondrial dissection technique for rhinoplasty with management of the nasal ligaments. Aesthet Surg J 2012;32(5):564–74.
10. Ozmen S, Eryilmaz T, Sencan A, et al. Sliding alar cartilage (SAC) flap: a new technique for nasal tip surgery. Ann Plast Surg 2009;63(5):480–5.
11. Gruber RP, Zhang AY, Zang A, et al. Preventing alar retraction by preservation of the lateral crus. Plast Reconstr Surg 2010;126(2):581–8.
12. Davis RE. Lateral crural tensioning for refinement of the wide and underprojected nasal tip: rethinking the lateral crural steal. Facial Plast Surg Clin North Am 2015;23(1):23–53.
13. Saban Y, Daniel RK, Polselli R, et al. Dorsal preservation: the push down technique reas- sessed. Aesthet Surg J 2018;38(2):117–31.
14. Çakır B, Küçüker İ, Aksakal İA, et al. Auto-Rim Flap Technique for Lateral Crura Caudal Excess Treatment. Aesthet Surg J 2017;37(1):24–32. PMID: 27694454.
15. Cakir B. Aesthetic Septorhinoplasty. 2nd Edition. Budapest: Springer; 2022.
16. Finocchi V, Vellone V, Mattioli RG, et al. A 3-Level Impaction Technique for Dorsal Reshaping and Reduction Without Dorsal Soft Tissue Envelope Dissection. Aesthet Surg J 2022;42(2):151–65.
17. Ishida LC, Ishida J, Ishida LH, et al. Nasal Hump Treatment With Cartilaginous Push-Down and Preservation of the Bony Cap. Aesthet Surg J 2020; 40(11):1168–78.
18. Orak F, Baghaki S. Use of osseocartilaginous paste graft for refinement of the nasal dorsum in rhinoplasty. Aesthet Plast Surg 2013;37(5):876–81.
19. Robotti E, Chauke-Malinga NY, Leone F. A Modified Dorsal Split Preservation Technique for Nasal Humps with Minor Bony Component: A Preliminary Report. Aesthet Plast Surg 2019;43(5):1257–68.

Surface Techniques in Dorsal Preservation

Miguel Gonçalves Ferreira, MD, PhD[a],*, Mariline Santos, MD[b]

KEYWORDS

- rhinoplasty • preservation • dorsum • surface techniques

KEY POINTS

- preservation rhinoplasty, surface techniques, dorsal modulation, Spare Roof Technique A, Spare Roof Technique B, Ferreira - Ishida Technique, Ishida Technique, Septorhinoplasty by Disarticulation, Cartilage-Only Pushdown

INTRODUCTION

In the 1990s, 4 decades after Cottle's introduction of the push-down concept for dorsal preservation (DP), Ishida described a new concept—dorsal modulation: splitting the osseous and cartilaginous middle vaults with the aims of preserving the cartilaginous middle vault integrity while simultaneously avoiding fracture impaction of the nasal pyramid.[1] This second technique addresses the main concern, which is the unpredictability associated with the "impaction fractures" maneuvers.

Today, DP is a complex area of rhinoplasty due to the number of new techniques and modifications that have been developed in recent years. Conceptually and structurally, there are 2 different groups in DP: the foundation techniques (FTs) and the surface techniques (STs).[2]

FTs are based on dorsal impaction, which involves impaction of the nasal pyramid into the face, requiring impaction osteotomies—push down or let down.[2]

STs are based on dorsal modulation, the hump is treated superficially with modulation of the middle vault, without impaction osteotomies—no bony push or let down.[2]

Over the years, several techniques for DP by dorsal modulation have been described in the literature. Examples:

Ishida (1999) Ishida Cartilaginous Push-Down (ICPD)

Jankowksi (2013) Septorhinoplasty by Disarticulation (SBD)

Ferreira (2016 and 2022) Spare Roof Technique— (SRT A and B)

Kosins (2017) Cartilage-Only Pushdown (COP)

This article will focus on these 4 STs, highlighting their similarities, differences, and how they have been overcoming some drawbacks previously reported with other surgical techniques frequently used in DP.

ISHIDA
Ishida Cartilaginous Pushdown

Procedure
The cartilaginous pushdown approach to nasal hump treatment is based on preserving and repositioning the cartilaginous portion of the hump while treating the bony portion with conventional osteotomies (**Fig. 1**).[1,3]

Conflict of Interest: The authors declare that they have no conflict of interest.
Compliance with Ethical Standards: Ethical approval: All opinions are in accordance with the ethical standards of the institutional and national research committee and with the 1964 Helsinki declaration and its later amendments or comparable ethical standards.
FINANCIAL DISCLOSURE: The authors declare that they have no financial disclosure to declare.
ª Centro Hospitalar Universitário do Porto, Instituto de Ciências Biomédicas Abel Salazar – Universidade do Porto, Hospital da Luz – Arrábida, Clínica do Nariz e Face, Porto, Portugal; ᵇ Centro Hospitalar Universitário do Porto, Instituto de Ciências Biomédicas Abel Salazar – Universidade do Porto, Porto, Portugal
* Corresponding author. R Dr. Miguel Martins, 282, Matosinhos 4450-806, Portugal.
E-mail address: mgferreira.md@gmail.com

Facial Plast Surg Clin N Am 31 (2023) 45–57
https://doi.org/10.1016/j.fsc.2022.08.005

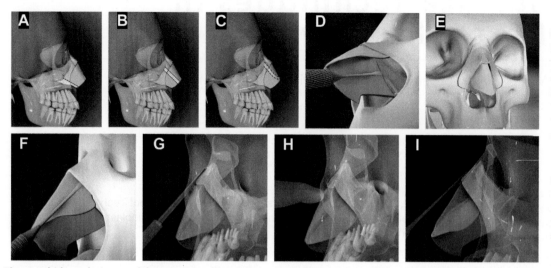

Fig. 1. Ishida technique— (*A*) Low strip, (*B*) medium strip, (*C*) high strip, (*D*) disarticulation of the septum/ethmoid, (*E*) final aspect after lateral osteotomies, (*F*) dissection of lateral keystone area, (*G*) triangular dorsal osteotomies, (*H*) cartilaginous pushdown, and (*I*) rasp of the remaining bone after the pushdown.

A strip of septal cartilage is resected parallel to the dorsum, preferably at the more deviated portion of the septal cartilage, which in most deviations tends to occur at the base of the septal cartilage, near the palatal crest. When septal deviation is absent or minimal, the preferred spot for resection is approximately 3 to 4 mm below the dorsum. The high septal strip preserves the caudal portion of the septal cartilage, which may be of use when treating difficult nasal tips.

The upper lateral cartilages (ULCs) are freed from the nasal bones using a Freer dissector, beginning close to the keystone area (see **Fig. 1**). The lateral length of dissection between the ULCs and the osseous pyriform aperture will determine how far the dorsum will be lowered, and this dissection should therefore be performed incrementally. The stability of the middle third depends on the remaining attachments between the ULCs and the nasal bones alongside the fibrous connective tissues (pyriform ligament) including the sesamoids. The septal cartilage is then completely detached from the perpendicular plate of the ethmoid (PPE) to mobilize the cartilaginous hump (see **Fig. 1**).

The bony cap is either resected or preserved, as described by Ishida in 2020.[3] To preserve the bony cap, 2 osteotomies are performed in the keystone area: beginning just short of the widest point in the middle third of the nose and converging to the midline at halfway up the nasal bones length. This bony cap in the keystone area will be lowered together with the cartilaginous portion of the hump (see **Fig. 1**). The residual lateral bony hump is then rasped to the desired level. The lateral

osteotomies bring the nasal bones closer to the midline and further help stabilize the cartilaginous hump in place. Medial osteotomies are performed as needed.

JANKOWSKI
Septorhinoplasty by Disarticulation

Procedure
SBD allows for the correction of septopyramidal deformities resulting from natural growth conflicts between nasal septum and pyramid.[4] Growing conflicts are first released at the septum level by the following:

1. Complete disarticulation of the anterior, inferior, and posterior edges of the quadrangular cartilage from the columella, vomer bone, and PPE, respectively, preserving the attachments of the superior edge of the quadrangular cartilage.
2. Enlarging the septal bony frame of the quadrangular cartilage by piecemeal resection of the vomer and lower half of the perpendicular plate, preserving respectively the choanal edge of the vomer and the upper half of the perpendicular plate under the cribriform plate. The upper limit of perpendicular plate resection follows from nasal bone tip to upper edge of the sphenoid rostrum.
3. Adjusting the quadrangular cartilage size by on demand resection of the anterior, inferior, and posterior edges of the quadrangular cartilage while preserving as much cartilage as possible of the quadrangular plate.

Following these disarticulation maneuvers, (1) the long-lasting elasticity of the quadrangular cartilage restores the flat surface of the remaining quadrangular plate and (2) the septolateral cartilages, hanging attached to the roof are rotated downward into the septal pocket, producing a retro-lobular saddling at the level of the cartilaginous dorsum, which is corrected by pulling on and replacing the antero-inferior edge of the quadrangular cartilage onto the premaxilla bone.[5]

When a simple septoplasty is being performed in case of a straight dorsum that needs no correction. In cases with a nasal hump and/or a deviated bony dorsum needing correction, the fibrocartilaginous nose (formed from alar and septolateral cartilages connected and to the skull base by ligaments of the olfactory fascia) is disarticulated subperiosteally beneath the bony dorsum from the tip of the piriform aperture to the nasion.[6] The periosteum is elevated on the superior aspect of the bony dorsum too. Resection of the bony hump through an open approach is followed by 2 paramedian osteotomies to the nasion to completely disarticulate the lateral slopes at their upper medial limit. Lateral osteotomies disarticulating their inferior limit in the basal sulcus of the frontal process of the maxillary bone are performed through nasal vestibular incisions. Thereafter, the posterior edge of each lateral slopes can usually easily be broken transcutaneously. The freed lateral slopes are then repositioned. By pulling on and replacing onto the premaxilla the antero-inferior edge of the rectified quadrangular cartilage, the full length of the fibrocartilaginous arch attached to the nasion and skull base becomes naturally straight to support the freed lateral slopes. If needed, tip surgery using classic techniques is performed at this stage.

Trans-columella sutures through the anterior edge of the quadrangular cartilage can be used to reposition it on the premaxilla and are knotted atop a bolster placed under the columella.

FERREIRA
Spare Roof Technique—SRT A and B

The spare roof technique (SRT) is a DP technique, described in 2016 by Ferreira MG and colleagues, which allows the surgeon to isolate the cartilaginous roof of the middle third without splitting the ULCs among them.[7]

SRT-A includes ostectomy of the bony cap.[7–9] However, considering the clinical and surgical experience acquired during the past years, for patients with V-shaped nasal bones (VSNB) and up to medium S-shaped nasal bones (SSNB), it would be possible to dehump the nose while preserving

the dorsal keystone area (DKA). Thus, based on rational anatomic basis, and the acquired experience with SRT-A, described by Ferreira MG and colleagues,[7–10] and cartilaginous push-down with preservation of the bony cap, described by Ishida LC and colleagues,[1,3] the authors designed a new technique for reduction rhinoplasty. This new technique named "spare roof technique B" or "Ferreira-Ishida technique" preserves the bony cap and ensures intact brow-tip dorsal esthetic lines.[11]

SRT-B

Procedure
The SRT-B can be performed by closed or open approach and includes 5 main steps:

Step 1 The architecture of this technique is based on the ideal dorsal esthetic lines. Thus, one must start by drawing on the surface of the skin, with the patient awake (**Fig. 2**):

- The desired dorsal brow-tip esthetic lines.
- The caudal limit of the nasal and maxillary bones—pyriform aperture.
- The Rhinion and the amount of triangular bone that will be necessary to take out to allow pushing-down the bony cap.
- The transversal line in the beginning of the nasal hump (in the cephalo-caudal direction).

Step 2 Lateral Walls:

By using the endonasal approach, bone cuts (ultrasonic) are performed. The paramedian high parallel osteotomies are performed exactly below the marked brow-tip dorsal esthetic lines. Then, perform the second group of lower osteotomies, till the cephalic level of the E-point, to achieve a triangular shape of bone in each side of the bony cap.

Perform the ostectomy of the mentioned triangular areas.

Release the lateral keystone area (LKA) with a Cottle dissector as needed.[12]

Step 3 Central compartment (**Fig. 3**):

With a #15 blade or scissor, release the ULCs from the dorsal septum: from the E-point[10] to the anterior nasal end of the ULCs (W-point),[12] immediately below the ULCs, separating completely the dorsal aspect of the septum from the ULCs, preserving the union among the ULCs (which remain preserved)—"high strip approach."

Excision of the longitudinal cartilage strip, from the E-Point till the W-Point (see **Fig. 2**). The highness of this strip is superior to the amount that one wants do decrease the hump.

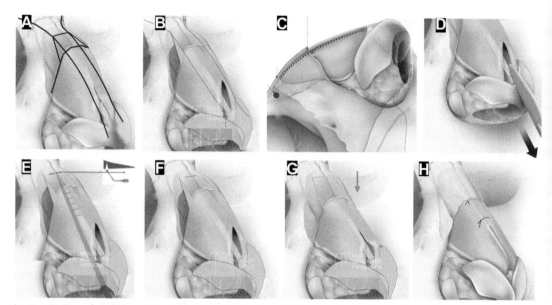

Fig. 2. Spare roof technique B—(*A*) Design of the desired dorsal esthetic lines—DALs, (*B*) triangular ostectomy immediately out of the DALs plus dissection of the LKA, (*C, D*) subdorsal strip from the E-point to the W-point, (*E*) subdorsal palisade cut plus subdorsal ostectomy, (*F, G*) gentle greenstick fracture—final pushdown, and (*H*) suture the cartilaginous middle vault to the septum with 5 to 0 PDS.

The remaining 1 to 2 mm of septum that stays attached to the cartilaginous middle vault must be scored with very light palisade cuts—#15 blade.

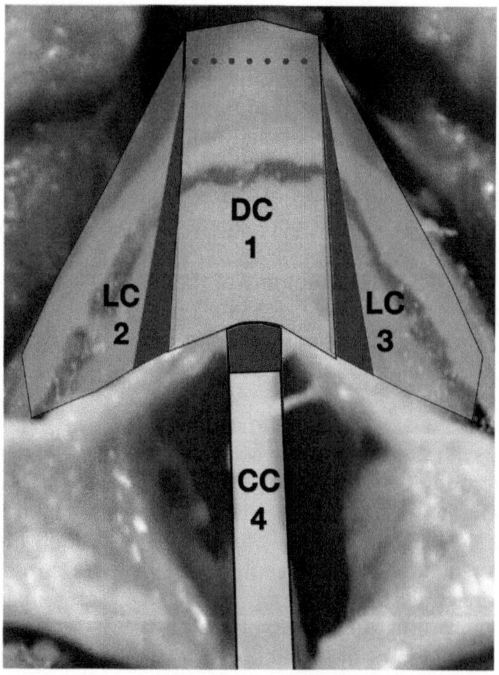

Fig. 3. Structure expresses only in the vertical compartments (2 lateral and the central) sparing completely the dorsal compartment.

The subdorsal osteotomy—perform partial transverse ostectomy (ultrasonic) on the undersurface of the nasal bones, right on the middle of the nose, in the sagittal plane just starting in the E-point in direction of the Selion.[13] This will allow to weaken the nasal bones and the posterior greenstick fracture.

Gently, push down the rectangular bony cap with your thumb or any smooth forceps in a greenstick fashion.

Perform lateral traditional osteotomies high–low–high to narrow the bony bridge as much as you need. We recommend endonasal osteotomies with previous subperiosteal dissection to create a tunnel access.

Step 4 Perform a regular L-shape Cottle septoplasty (when necessary).

Step 5 Perform the suture of the cartilaginous middle vault (ULCs) to the dorsal aspect of the remaining septum, just after the Rhinion (in the cephalocaudal direction), with absorbable polydioxanone 5 to 0, to stabilize the roof and fix any spring effect that might still exists. It is easier to perform it by open approach. For closed approach, we developed the "Hump-Apex Suture": a guided suture through the skin and middle vault. It includes 4 main steps: Step 1—pass the suture through the middle of the septum in a point vertical to the Rhinion. After this, one will have the 2 ends of the suture in each side of the septum.

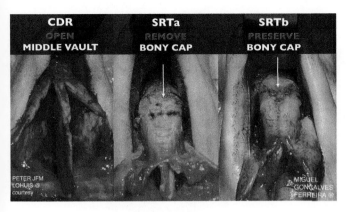

Fig. 4. Sequence of techniques that the surgeon MGF has used for till the moment.

Step 2—introduce an #18 Abocath in the highest point of the hump, immediately after the Rhinion, through the skin plus ULCs till the left side and insert the left end of the suture through the lumen of the Abocath. Step 3—pull the Abocath up the ULCs but remain below the skin, and move it gently to the opposite side. Then, enter it again thorough the ULCs and do the same procedure with the right end of the suture. Step 4—pull the Abocath (with both ends of the suture) out of the skin and tie the knot of this suture through the skin hole—not attached to the skin. Finally, release the dorsal skin from the knot.

Advantages SRT-B is faster than SRT-A and the traditional structured procedures (**Fig. 4**) because it is not necessary to uncap the bony hump, and/or reconstruct the middle vault, either with spreader grafts or spreader flaps. Esthetically, the dorsum is smoother, and the absence of grafts or flaps is much more likely to avoid dorsal defects in the medium and long-term results.

The advantages of the spare roof technique (A and B) over the classic push/let down are supported by some rational reasons:

a. Esthetic and functional outcomes tested and published:[9,14]

The first prospective study with the highest level of evidence ever published in "Preservation Rhinoplasty" until 2020 was published in 2019 on this technique.[9]

b. Stability of the keystone area tested and published:[9,14]

With this technique, the stability of the middle vault was tested and is reliable as expected, despite all theoretic doubts on the stability after releasing the LKA. The concerns about the stability of LKA when it is "touched" are based on the traditional "structured techniques"[9] in which the middle vault is opened and loses its architectural stability. In the SRT, all these structural mechanisms are preserved.

c. Efficient in crooked noses.[15]

"As the septum goes, so goes the nose." The first step of the SRT is exactly the splitting of these 2 structures—septum and ULCs. After performing this maneuver, typically, the cartilaginous crooked nose is immediately reallocated to the midline, and the nose is not crooked anymore. After that, we have a straight nose and a crooked septum, at that moment one decides what to do with the crooked septum—from minimal maneuvers till the extracorporeal septoplasty (**Figs. 5–8**).

d. Efficient in S-Shaped nasal bones.

e. Allows traditional septal maneuvers:

The traditional "L-shape" septoplasty is always performed. Any typical septal maneuver can be done.

f. Short learning curve:

Easy to split from "structured techniques" because this is a "transition technique," with some concepts similar to some "structured concepts."

g. Safe and predictable:

Medium-term and long-term results tend to be more predictable because there is no impaction of the bony and cartilaginous pyramid (**Figs. 9–14**).

KOSINS
Cartilage-Only Pushdown

Procedure
High septal strip After elevating the soft tissue envelope (STE), a wide submucosal dissection of the subdorsal septum is performed as well as dissecting for at least 5 mm under the ULCs.[16] Two anatomic points must be clearly delineated—anterior septal angle (ASA) and W-point.

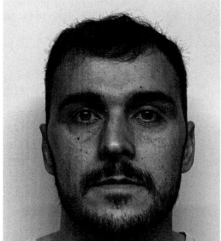 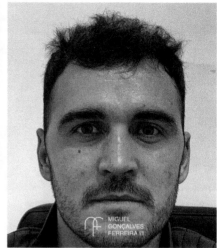

Fig. 5. Frontal view - SRT B in the crocked nose—pictures before and 12 months after surgery.

Cartilage-only high septal strip DP is a hybrid technique that consists of 4 steps:

1. modification/ostectomy of the bony cap including the LKA to convert the bony dorsum to cartilage.
2. high septal strip resection under the dorsum.
3. precise fixation of the cartilaginous vault to the underlying septum.
4. piezoelectric rhinosculpture and osteotomies to narrow and to sculpt the bony pyramid.

Thus, only the cartilaginous vault is lowered. The bones are dealt with separately and no impaction of the osseocartilaginous vault into the pyriform aperture is performed. Alternatively (as described by Ishida), in step 1, the surgeon may preserve

the bony cap and release it from the surrounding bone with paramedian osteotomies that are connected cephalically with a transverse osteotomy.[3] If the bony cap is flat, it can be preserved and lowered with the cartilage vault. If it is curved (convex), it is better to remove the bony cap or modify it for lowering along with the cartilage vault.

Step 1
Bony vault modification As previously described, there is no bony hump on the dorsum.[17] Rather, a *bony cap* exists that overlaps the cartilaginous vault. If the bone is convex, it can be removed incrementally, thereby exposing the underlying cartilaginous vault. This maneuver changes the proportions of the dorsum by increasing the

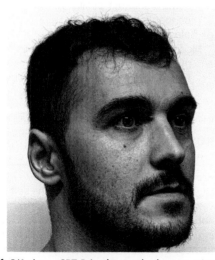 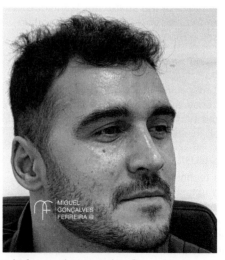

Fig. 6. Left 3/4 view - SRT B in the crocked nose—pictures before and 12 months after surgery.

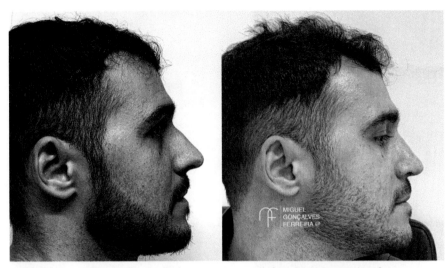

Fig. 7. Left Porfile view - SRT B in the crocked nose—pictures before and 12 months after surgery.

amount of exposed cartilage while removing excess bone. This procedure helps to create a more flexible osseocartilaginous joint and to decrease the convexity/kyphosis of the nasal profile. Bone is removed until the cephalic profile (area above the caudal end of the nasal bones) fits the desired postoperative profile. After incremental cap removal, only the cartilage must be lowered.

Step 2
High septal strip resection As in traditional DP, the initial strip resection starts approximately 8 to 10 mm cephalic to the ASA at the W-point. Initially, only 1.5 to 2 mm of septum is resected directly under the dorsum. This initial cut is done to break the tension of the osseocartilaginous joint. Curved scissors are used for the anterior cut to stay immediately under the dorsum and straight scissors for the posterior cut to ensure a straight cut. Any remaining septum on the undersurface of the osseocartilaginous vault can be scored with scissors to help further break the tension of the chondro-osseous joint. No PPE is removed as bony impaction is *not* part of this technique.

Step 3
Suture fixation of dorsum The cartilaginous vault is now sewn down to the underlying septum. Two 25-gauge needles are used to pin the cartilaginous vault in place. Then, sutures are used to secure the natural dorsum down into its new desired position. Sutures are placed from each shoulder of the ULC down to the underlying septum independently. In this way, the

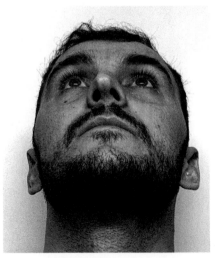
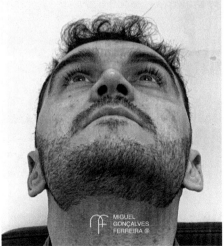

Fig. 8. Base view - SRT B in the crocked nose—pictures before and 12 months after surgery.

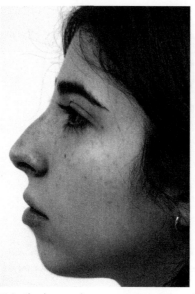
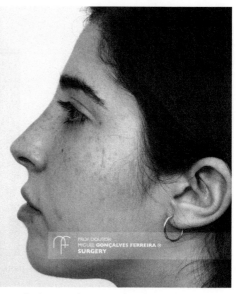

Fig. 9. SRT B in the humped nose and thin skin—pictures before and 12 months after surgery.

cartilaginous vault width and shape can be modified incrementally. If more than 2 mm of reduction is required, the cartilaginous vault must sometimes be partially released from the LKA to allow descent. Only enough LKA release is done to allow fixation. The ULCs are assessed for stiffness because stiffer cartilage requires more release from the LKA.

Step 4
Refining the bony pyramid After the cartilaginous profile is lowered to the point of harmony

with the bony vault. This lowering of the cartilage vault will create the dorsal and lateral esthetic lines. No open roof deformity needs to be closed because the middle vault has been maintained. In this way, the lateral bone is treated separately from the cartilaginous vault that remains intact. It should be noted that narrowing/modification of the bony vault can be easily done with traditional instruments but piezoelectric instrumentation and the full open approach makes uncapping and osteotomies easier and more predictable.[18]

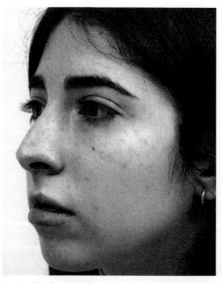
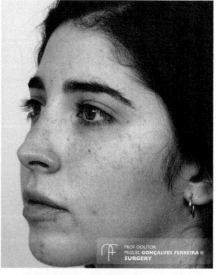

Fig. 10. SRT B in the humped nose and thin skin—pictures before and 12 months after surgery.

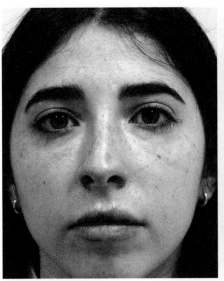
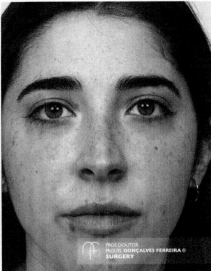

Fig. 11. SRT B in the humped nose and thin skin—pictures before and 12 months after surgery.

DISCUSSION
Why Surface Techniques?

Anatomic considerations
The 2 most important anatomic landmarks/concepts in STs are the E-point and V-shaped or S-shaped nasal bones:

1. The E-point introduced by Ferreira and colleagues[10] represents the point where the PPE meets the undersurface of the nasal bones and is crucial in the concept of the SRT. The authors have studied their population and found that 97% of the nasal humps begin caudally to the E-Point. In most cases, the hump is therefore not supported by the PPE, highlighting that it is very rare the need to touch the PPE while dehumping.

2. In the Caucasian humped nose, there are 2 main types of nasal bone configuration: first, the SSNB introduced by Lazovic and colleagues,[19] accounting in this study for the vast majority (88%), and second, the VSNB. The SSNB have a Kyphotic configuration, which means that the caudal aspect of the nasal bones is convex in such a way that it is virtually impossible to correct with traditional

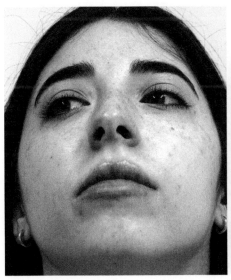
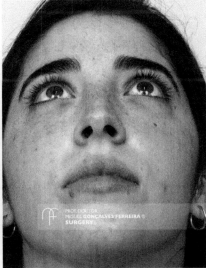

Fig. 12. SRT B in the humped nose and thin skin—pictures before and 12 months after surgery.

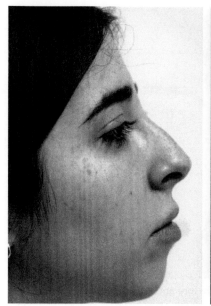
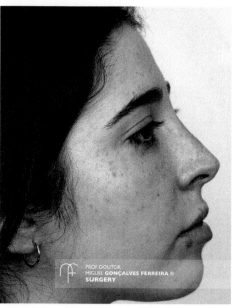

Fig. 13. SRT B in the humped nose and thin skin—pictures before and 12 months after surgery.

push/let down techniques. The only efficient way to flatten a significantly kyphotic bony hump is by performing ostectomy, as performed in SBD, SRT-A or COP—the so called dorsal modulation.

No impaction osteotomies
The total absence of impaction osteotomies results in more predictable results.

All the techniques to dehump—either structured or preservation—have, somewhere, a triangular ostectomy as one of the most important steps.

Due to the geometric proprieties of the nasal pyramid/hump, in STs—structured or preservation—the triangular ostectomy is smaller than in FTs—this led to higher unpredictability in FTs.

WHAT ARE THE SIMILARITIES AND DIFFERENCES AMONG SUPERFICIAL TECHNIQUES FOR DORSAL PRESERVATION?

In **Fig. 15**, similarities and differences among these 4 techniques are summarized.

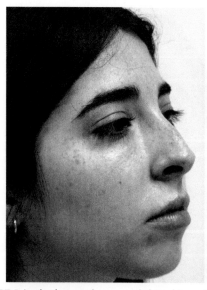
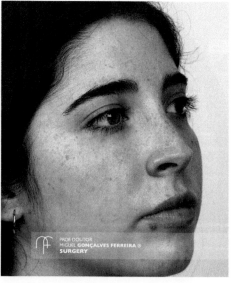

Fig. 14. SRT B in the humped nose and thin skin—pictures before and 12 months after surgery.

PRESERVATION RHINOPLASTY - SURFACE TECHNIQUES				
	ISHIDA *ICPD* 1999	**JANKOVSKY** *SBD* 2013	**FERREIRA** *SRT a & b* 2016/20	**KOSINS** *COP* 2017
CARTILAGINOUS MIDDLE VAULT	PRESERVED	PRESERVED	PRESERVED	PRESERVED
DORSAL BONY CAP	PRESERVED triangular	REMOVED	PRESERVED quadrangular DAL's	REMOVED
SEPTAL STRIP	HIGH / MEDIUM LOW	LOW	SUBDORSAL	SUBDORSAL
SEPTOPLASTY	SWINGING DOOR	SWINGING DOOR	L-SHAPE	L-SHAPE
ULCs/SEPTUM SUTURE	YES	NO	YES	YES
ETHMOID PRESERVED	YES	NO	YES	YES

Fig. 15. Similarities and differences among 4 superficial techniques for dorsal preservation.

INDICATIONS

The indications for these techniques are patients with a dorsal hump without previous rhinoplasty by component dorsal reduction.

In primary and in secondary rhinoplasties with the ULCs intact, there is no contraindication. After passing the learning curve, one will find these techniques suitable to approach virtually any primary rhinoplasty.

The crooked nose is also elective.[15]

In the end, all noses that still have the "roof" are eligible for STs.

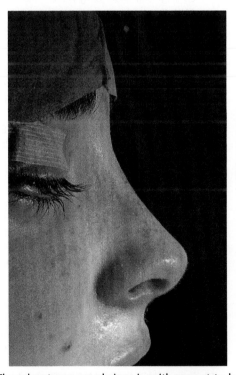 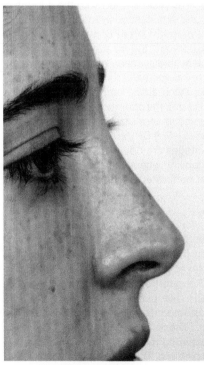

Fig. 16. The advantages are obvious in with respect to healing and predictability whenever the dorsum is not dissected or perforated.

CONTRAINDICATIONS

For COP, Kosins and colleagues describe a limitation for humps larger than 3.5 mm. The authors wrote that these large humps are *not* done routinely with this technique because a large amount of release/disarticulation is required, which can be destabilizing and allow for more irregularity on the dorsum.

For SRT-B, the only major contraindication is the severe SSNB, in which it becomes impossible to flatten the bony kyphosis without doing some degree of ostectomy—SRT-A. The size of the hump is not a contraindication for the SRT-B.

BONY CAP—PRESERVE OR REMOVE?

It seems logical that the bony cap preservation minimizes the irregularities over the keystone area while performing the cartilaginous pushdown. After this preservation, there is no need for any type of dorsal camouflage.

The preservation of the bony cap does not impede lateral and paramedial medial osteotomies, allowing the bony pyramid to be narrowed when necessary.

FULL DORSAL PRESERVATION—NO DISSECTION OF THE DORSUM

When the SRT-B is performed with the subdorsal osteotomy, and simultaneously there is no relevant deformity/asymmetry in the bony or cartilaginous part of the dorsum, the operation is performed with absolutely no dissection of the nasal dorsum.

In most of the primary rhinoplasties, where a smooth and symmetric hump is the only issue (no matter its size), the operation is done with complete preservation of all layers inside the dorsal esthetical lines—Full DP.

The advantages are obvious in terms of healing and predictability whenever the dorsum is not dissected or perforated (**Fig. 16**).

SUMMARY

Preservation STs, as structured techniques, theoretically allow more precision because the surgeon is operating exactly "in" the problem and still maintains the 3D support of the nasal pyramid.

Classic DP rhinoplasty is typically done with impaction osteotomies (push/let down) and a low septal strip. These approaches are potentially highly destabilizing maneuvers in the architecture of the nasal pyramid. This is for sure one of the reasons why these approaches did not have a popular acceptance in the 1960s and 1970s.

More recently, the surgeon interested in preservation rhinoplasty has the possibility to do so with STs with more control and easily convertible to the standard structured techniques whenever the surgeon does not feel safe with the procedure.

REFERENCES

1. Ishida J, Ishida LC, Ishida LH, et al. Treatment of the nasal hump with preservation of the cartilaginous framework. Plast Reconstr Surg 1999;103(6): 1729–35.
2. Gonçalves Ferreira M, Toriumi DM. A Practical Classification System for Dorsal Preservation Rhinoplasty Techniques. Facial Plast Surg Aesthet Med 2021; 23(3):153–5.
3. Ishida LC, Ishida J, Ishida LH, et al. Nasal Hump Treatment With Cartilaginous Push-Down and Preservation of the Bony Cap. Aesthet Surg J 2020; 40(11):1168–78.
4. Jankowski R. Septoplastie et Rhinoplastie par Désarticulation. Paris: Elsevier Masson; 2016.
5. Varoquier M, Rumeau C, Vuissoz PA, et al. Do the upper lateral nasal cartilages exist? The concept of septolateral cartilages. Eur Ann Otorhinolaryngol Head Neck Dis 2021;138(2):77–81.
6. Jankowski R, Rumeau C, de Saint Hilaire T, et al. The olfactory fascia: an evo-devo concept of the fibrocartilaginous nose. Surg Radiol Anat 2016;38(10): 1161–8.
7. Ferreira MG, Monteiro D, Reis C, et al. Spare Roof Technique: A Middle Third New Technique. Facial Plast Surg 2016;32(1):111–6.
8. Gonçalves Ferreira M, Santos M, Rosa F, et al. Spare Roof Technique: A New Technique for Hump Removal-The Step-by-Step Guide. Plast Reconstr Surg 2020;145(2):403–6.
9. Santos M, Rego ÂR, Coutinho M, et al. Spare roof technique in reduction rhinoplasty: Prospective study of the first one hundred patients. Laryngoscope 2019;129(12):2702–6.
10. Ferreira MG, Dias DR, Cardoso L, et al. Dorsal Hump Reduction Based on the New Ethmoidal Point Classification: A Clinical and Radiological Study of the Keystone Area in 138 Patients. Aesthet Surg J 2020;40(9):950–9.
11. Gonçalves Ferreira M, Ishida LC, Ishida LH, et al. Ferreira-Ishida Technique: Spare Roof Technique B. Step-by-Step Guide to Preserving the Bony Cap While Dehumping. Plast Reconstr Surg 2022; 149(5):901e–4e.
12. Daniel RK, Pálházi P. Osteocartilaginous Vault. Rhinoplasty: an anatomical and clinical atlas. New York, NY: Springer International Publishing; 2018.
13. Ferreira MG, Santos M, Dias D. Subdorsal Osteotomy and Complete Dorsal Preservation - A New

Paradigm in Preservation Rhinoplasty? Laryngoscope 2022;132(4):769–71.

14. Ferreira MG, Santos M, E Carmo DO, et al. Spare Roof Technique Versus Component Dorsal Hump Reduction: A Randomized Prospective Study in 250 Primary Rhinoplasties, Aesthetic and Functional Outcomes. Aesthet Surg J 2021;41(3):288–300.

15. Rodrigues Dias D, Santos M, Sousa E Castro S, et al. The Spare Roof Technique as a New Approach to the Crooked Nose. Facial Plast Surg Aesthet Med 2022. https://doi.org/10.1089/fpsam.2021.0368 [published online ahead of print, 2022 Apr 11].

16. Kosins AM. Expanding Indications for Dorsal Preservation Rhinoplasty With Cartilage Conversion Techniques. Aesthet Surg J 2021;41(2):174–84.

17. Palhazi P, Daniel RK, Kosins AM. The osseocartilaginous vault of the nose: anatomy and surgical observations. Aesthet Surg J 2015;35(3):242–51.

18. Gerbault O, Daniel RK, Kosins AM. The Role of Piezoelectric Instrumentation in Rhinoplasty Surgery. Aesthet Surg J 2016;36(1):21–34.

19. Lazovic GD, Daniel RK, Janosevic LB, et al. Rhinoplasty: the nasal bones - anatomy and analysis. Aesthet Surg J 2015;35(3):255–63.

Open Preservation Rhinoplasty Using the Piezo Electric Instrument

Abdulkadir Goksel, MD*, Khanh Ngoc Tran, MBBS

KEYWORDS

- Rhinoplasty • Preservation rhinoplasty • Open rhinoplasty • Piezosurgery
- Piezo electric instrument

KEY POINTS

- Preservation rhinoplasty is more than just dorsal preservation—ligamentous and alar cartilage preservation are other critical elements.
- The Piezo device, with tips such as saws, rasps, scrapers, and drills, allows for precise management of the osseocartilaginous vault, enables delicate bone reshaping, the creation of osteotomies in specific planes to permit accurate bony vault lowering and tilting, and safe perforation of mobile nasal bones or the nasal spine for dorsal and septal fixation.
- For effective dorsal lowering, key blocking points causing potential resistance to dorsal lowering should be considered and if necessary addressed, including Webster's triangle excision, releasing the periosteum along the inner surface of the maxillary bone, and performing limited lateral nasal keystone release (Ballerina maneuver).

INTRODUCTION AND BACKGROUND

Achieving smooth and straight dorsal esthetic lines and obtaining predictable, long-lasting results are some of the most important albeit challenging aspects of rhinoplasty surgery. The most commonly used method to achieve dorsal lowering is through conventional hump resection using osteotomies and rasping; however, such techniques cause disruption of the keystone area, necessitating middle vault reconstruction or camouflage methods to counter any ensuing surface irregularities. Although reconstruction can achieve great results, even in the best hands it cannot bring back the natural anatomy. Therefore, the question arises that if there is the possibility for us to achieve a satisfactory esthetic and functional result while simultaneously preserving the patient's natural dorsal anatomy, then why should we create a defect that we would only need to repair later on? Why not instead reshape the nose by lowering the dorsal height while simultaneously preserving the nasal dorsal line? This is the philosophy behind preservation of rhinoplasty surgery.

The expression "preservation rhinoplasty" was first coined in a 2018 editorial by Daniel[1] to describe the three pillars of preservation surgery: dorsal, alar cartilage, and soft tissue/ligamentous preservation. Despite having a century-long history, widespread adoption of dorsal preservation techniques in the past was slow and oftentimes stagnated, particularly with the advent of open structural rhinoplasty.[2] Recently, however there has been a resurgence of interest in preservation techniques, resulting in critical modifications to existing maneuvers, the development of innovative new surgical methods, and the publication of several landmark articles and texts on this subject, making preservation rhinoplasty more accessible and appealing to a wider audience of surgeons.[1–3] Furthermore, the introduction of innovative powered surgical instruments such as the Piezo-electric device are considered by many to be a welcome addition to the surgical

Rinolstanbul Facial Plastic Surgery Clinic, Istanbul 34738, Turkey
* Corresponding author. Bagdat Cad. No:378/5 Sakinbakkal Kadikoy, Istanbul, Turkey
E-mail address: akgoksel@gmail.com

Facial Plast Surg Clin N Am 31 (2023) 59–71
https://doi.org/10.1016/j.fsc.2022.08.007

toolbox,[4] as they enable easier and more accurate reshaping of the bony dorsum as well as the creation of more delicate, precise and controlled osteotomies for "let down" and "push down" procedures when lowering the bony vault in dorsal preservation surgery.

In this article, we detail the various preservation rhinoplasty techniques that enable dorsal modification and preservation. We outline the indications and applications, describing the various advantages as well as the potential difficulties that may be encountered. Particular emphasis is given to complication prevention measures and important technical points. We will also be discussing limited soft tissue dissection techniques, with the preservation of the ligamentous attachments and the benefits of doing so. It is our preference to perform these operations through an open approach with the assistance of Piezo-electric instruments (PEI), to provide better anatomic exposure and improved technical precision. Clinical examples of our open preservation cases using PEI can be seen in the following before (**Figs. 1**A–E and **2A–E**) and after (**Figs.** 1F–J and **2F–J**) patient photographs.

DISCUSSION
Patient Selection

The main rhinoplasty indication in Caucasian patients, which constitutes the majority of our patients, is the nasal dorsal hump. When deciding whether a patient is suitable for dorsal preservation, it is essential for the surgeon to first assess the patient's dorsum and its deformity and decide whether they wish to preserve it.

Dorsal preservation is most ideally suited to primary cases where there are short v-shaped nasal bones, a predominantly cartilaginous small dorsal hump, high to normal radix, and straight dorsal esthetic lines with linear axis deviation.[3] Narrow tension noses are also suited to this technique. **Box 1** outlines the indications, according to the various septal techniques. In our practice, we consider contraindications to dorsal preservation to be the following: (1) difficult septoplasties (multiple fractures septum, large septal perforation, high septal or severe deviations), (2) when total or partial nasal septal reconstruction is required, (3) severe S-shaped axis deviations, (4) secondary cases, (5) patients with prior open roof reduction rhinoplasty, and (6) patients whose angle between the nasal bone and the upper lateral cartilages (ULCs) is less than 150°. Such cases are better managed using classical structure or hybrid techniques.

Having established patient suitability, the surgeon must then evaluate the severity and composition of the dorsal convexity, any deviated aspects of the bony and cartilaginous dorsum and the presence of any septal pathology, to determine the following key technical elements: (1) the surgical approach and extent of ligamentous preservation—preservation rhinoplasty can be performed via either open or closed approaches with varying plans for dorsal skin and ligamentous dissection; (2) management of the septum; (3) management of the dorsal osseocartilaginous vault; (4) whether ancillary procedures are needed to facilitate dorsal lowering, such as bony cap removal to convert an osseocartilaginous hump into a purely cartilaginous one, or dissection of the lateral keystone area (Goksel's Ballerina maneuver) to prevent tissue resistance to dorsal descent and hump recurrence; and (5) points of fixation to secure the mobilized osseocartilaginous vault to the underlying septum.

Ligamentous Preservation

It is possible to keep the ligaments intact in open preservation rhinoplasty and where possible in our practice we endeavor to do so. As the nasal ligaments are the main connection between the skin and the nasal skeleton, by preserving them we can reduce post-operative swelling, enable better, faster re-draping of the nasal skin envelope, and oftentimes retain the natural elasticity.[5,6] This is particularly relevant for thick-skinned rhinoplasty patients, for whom the re-establishment of contours can often be difficult, especially in the early postoperative period. In our experience, preservation of the ligamentous and skin attachments will help to create better contours in these patients.[6]

During the patient selection process, we divide the patients into three groups according to their soft tissue and dorsal deformity.

Group 1

These patients have good dorsal esthetics, V-shaped nasal bones and only need reduction of the dorsal profile line. In this group, it is possible to perform preservation rhinoplasty via an open approach with no skin elevation on the dorsum and at the same time to preserve virtually all the nasal ligaments (**Fig. 3**A–C).

Group 2

These patients have good dorsal esthetic lines yet require modifications due to the height of the bony hump. In this group, it is necessary to elevate the dorsal skin and partially dissect the ligaments **Fig. 4**(A–C). We approach the dorsum via tunnels created between the Deep Pitanguy and vertical

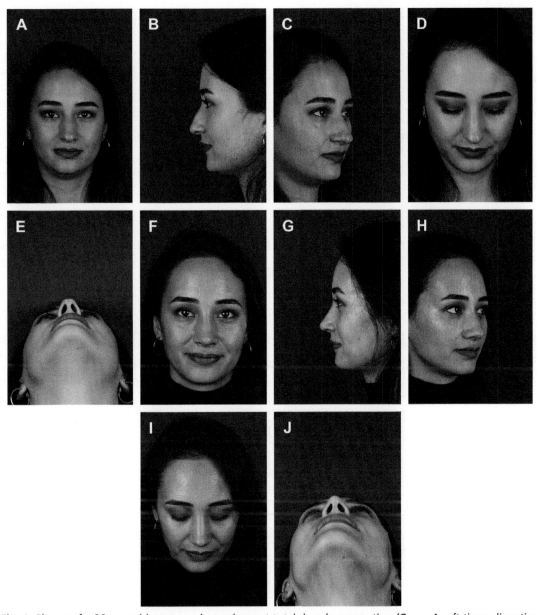

Fig. 1. Photos of a 26-year-old woman who underwent total dorsal preservation (Group 1 soft tissue dissection with complete ligamentous preservation) using Subdorsal septal flap technique and piezo-assisted symmetric sagittal low–low osteotomies. Preoperative (*A–E*) and 18 months postoperative (*F–J*) clinical photographs.

scroll ligament (VSL). With this maneuver, we can refine dorsal esthetic lines while still preserving the ligaments.

Group 3

In these patients, there are significant deformities on the dorsum; however, despite the existence of dorsal irregularities and asymmetries, dorsal preservation is still deemed feasible. In this group, the dorsum is reshaped and preserved through total dissection of the skin of the nasal dorsum

without any ligamentous preservation (**Fig. 5A–C**). The Pitanguy ligament and Scroll ligament can be fixed at the end of the procedure.

We can also preserve the nasomaxillary suture line ligament (NMSL),[6] delineated in **Fig. 6**, which is located along the suture line between the nasal bones and the frontal process of the maxilla, for the cases in Groups 1 and 2. It is an important structure when it comes to osteotomies, notably because if this ligament can be kept intact during the piezo osteotomies, in our experience skin redraping and healing will be faster. Preservation

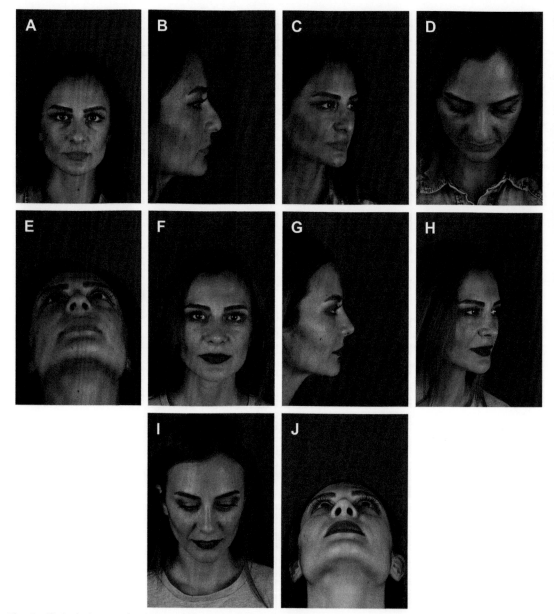

Fig. 2. Clinical photos of a 32-year-old woman who underwent total dorsal preservation (Group 1 soft tissue dissection with complete ligamentous preservation) with high-septal strip and piezo-assisted symmetric sagittal low–low osteotomies. Preoperative (*A–E*) and 12 months postoperative (*F–J*) photos.

of the NMS ligament can be achieved by creating a tunnel posterior to this ligament for the low-to-low osteotomies.

SURGICAL TECHNIQUE
Skin and Soft-Tissue Envelope Elevation

For the open approach, we prefer an inverted-V incision. For the skin and superficial musculoaponeurotic system (SMAS) dissection, it is crucial to first establish what is the planned procedure for

the nasal dorsum, as this will dictate the extent of soft tissue dissection.

Group 1: If we have no intended changes to make on the nasal dorsum, we continue with the ligament preservation method without dorsal skin dissection.

Group 2: For patients who need nasal dorsum reshaping by rasping or camouflage, we elevate the nasal skin supraperichondrially and dissect between the preserved VSL and Pitanguy's Ligaments. Some dorsums have S-shaped nasal

---

Box 1
Preservation rhinoplasty indications according to septal technique

High-septal strip approach

- Dorsal hump ≤4 mm
- Hump is mostly cartilaginous
- High-septal deviation
- Over-projected radix
- Caudal septum is in the midline
- Straight noses
- V shape nasal bones

Mid-Septal Strip/Subdorsal flap approach

- Same as high-septal strip (HSS)
- Slight crooked nose

Low-septal strip approach

- Same as HSS
- If there is pathology along the connection of the anterior nasal spine and maxillary crest with the septal cartilage
- Crooked nose with straight dorsal esthetic lines

Bony Dorsal Preservation

- Same as HSS
- Crooked nose with straight dorsal esthetic lines, where there is NO pathology at the septal base

---

bones,[7] in which case we dissect the bony dorsum in the subperiosteal plane for necessary rasping of the bony cap.

It is important to note that for during skin/SMAS dissection for Groups 1 and 2, we create a subperiosteal tunnel for lateral and transverse osteotomies by approaching the Pyriform Aperture via a rim incision just lateral to the VSL and the Pitanguy's Ligament, without nasal skin elevation. The lateral tunnel should be wide enough to enable the utilization of Piezo instruments under direct visualization.

Group 3: If there is a need for extensive reshaping on both the bony and cartilaginous dorsum, we cut through the Pitanguy's Ligament and the VSL, dissecting the skin in the supraperichondrial plane over the cartilaginous area and in the subperiosteal plane over the bony area. With a widened skin dissection, we extend the dissection to the radix area and pyriform aperture, including the superficial portion of the medial canthal ligament, which enables sufficient access for the use of Piezo instruments.

MANAGEMENT OF THE SEPTUM
Approaching the Septal Cartilage

In open preservation rhinoplasty cases where we intend to preserve all the ligaments, we reach the septal cartilage via a hemitransfixion incision. If we plan to cut the Pitanguy's ligament and make modifications on the nasal dorsum, we reach the septum through the caudal area without an additional incision. With regards to the septum, we recommend adopting the strategy described by

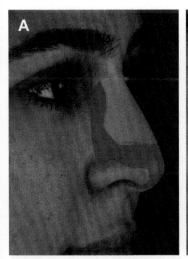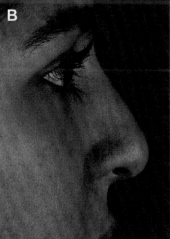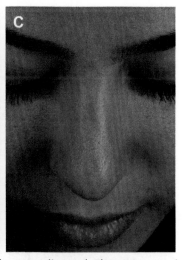

Fig. 3. (A–C). Group 1 Dissection. The red and orange zones represent the areas dissected. The green zone is intact, with no skin elevation.

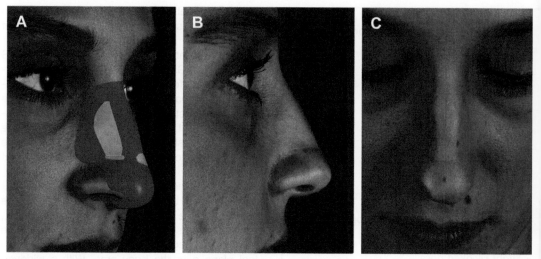

Fig. 4. (*A–C*). Group 2 Dissection. The red zone shows the dissected area. The green zone is not dissected and the skin is not elevated.

Neves,[8] whereby the septal cartilage is dissected in the supraperichondrial plane, otherwise referred to as the sublaminar plane as it lies below the lamina propria, in the regions where one intends to insert a suture to later fixate the dorsum. The intact perichondrial attachment to the septum affords additional strength to the septal cartilage and reduces the risk of suture material tearing through the cartilage upon dorsal fixation. For example, with low-septal strip techniques, we recommend that at least the most caudal 1 cm of septal cartilage be elevated in supraperichondrial plane, before switching to the bloodless subperichondrial plane for the remainder of the septal dissection. If the surgeon intends to place an adjacent septal graft (eg, septal extension graft, bony or

cartilaginous splint graft), we advise that on the side of intended grafting that the septum be elevated in a subperichondrial plane; however, on the non-graft side the perichondrium be kept intact in the regions of intended suture fixation.

Septal Strip Excision

Before osseocartilaginous pyramid mobilization, it is necessary to first create space for dorsal hump lowering, by resecting a septal strip. The main determinant of nasal dorsum lowering is not the amount of bone resected but the amount of septal strip removed. There are several established dorsal preservation septal maneuvers available, as illustrated in **Fig. 7**(A–G). They can be grouped

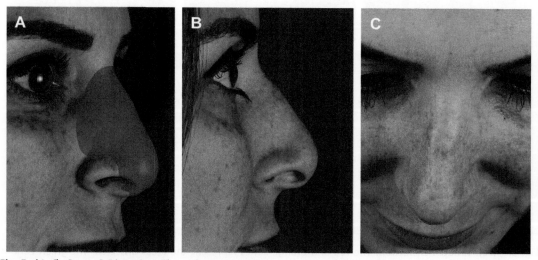

Fig. 5. (*A–C*). Group 3 Dissection. The red zone represents the area of dissection.

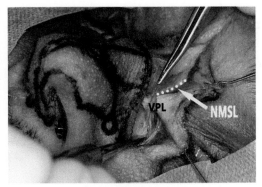

Fig. 6. The dotted line shows the nasomaxillary suture line ligament (NMSL) on the suture line between the frontal process of the maxillary bone and the nasal bone. VPL: vertical pyriform ligament.

into the following categories: (1) High-septal strip/subdorsal resection (as popularized by Saban[3]); (2) Mid-Septal Strip/Subdorsal flaps of various configurations (as per Most,[9] Neves[10] and Kovacevic[11]); (3) low-septal strip (Cottle[12] or Finocchi's[13] "SPQR" Simplified Preservation Quick Rhinoplasty/modified Cottle); and (4) Bony Dorsal Preservation (Goksel).[14]

Factors influencing the choice of septal procedure include (1) the surgeon's experience and the technique that he/she is best accustomed to; (2) presence of septal deviation, its location and severity; (3) whether the bony pyramid is deviated (crooked nose); and (4) other indications as previously outlined in **Box 1**.

MANAGEMENT OF THE BONY VAULT
Piezo Osteotomy/Ostectomy

PEI have been used for a long time in maxillofacial surgery and dentistry and have been shown to be a precise and safe surgical instrument with good applicability in rhinoplasty.[4] Thanks to the new generation of the devices, procedures such as reshaping, cutting through and rasping of the bones can be carried out much faster and with greater ease. Furthermore, PEI preserves the integrity of the surrounding soft tissues and membranes and does not cause significant bleeding during the bone shaping process, thereby drastically reducing both postoperative bleeding and edema.[4,15,16] This technique helps to avoid unwanted fracture lines and irregularities resulting from palpable bony spicules that usually occur with osteotomies carried out with osteotomes. Moreover, bone sculpting with PEI is possible even after bony vault mobilization. Gerbault's publication on Piezo surgery is an important resource for this subject.[4,15]

Addressing the Bony Vault

There are two main ways to manage the bony vault in DPR—the let-down and the push-down procedure. In both instances, the whole bony vault is

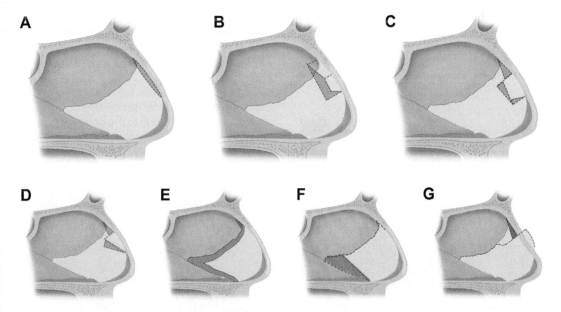

Fig. 7. Preservation septal maneuvers. (A) Saban high-septal strip; Subdorsal flap variations include (B) most subdorsal flap, (C) neves tetris flap, (D) Kovacevic Z-Flap; low-septal techniques include (E) Cottle low-septal strip and (F) Finocchi SPQR; (G) goksel bony dorsal preservation.

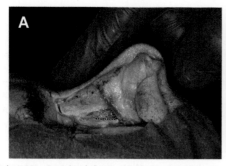
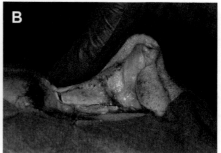

Fig. 8. Webster's triangle. (*A*) in relation to lateral osteotomy, (*B*) following resection and push down.

mobilized and lowered using lateral, transverse, and radix osteotomies. If a strip of bone is resected laterally at the facial groove and the bony pyramid descends to sit on the ascending frontal process of the maxilla, this is known as a let-down. If however, following osteotomies, the bony pyramid is impacted down into the pyriform aperture with bony overlap, this is called a push-down.

In our practice we use piezoelectric instruments for all our lateral bone osteotomies; they enable us to create delicate osteotomies at a more precise level and change the direction of the bony cuts from horizontal to sagittal, thus decreasing the bony resistance to posterior displacement during push-down. In both let-down and the push-down cases, we conduct low-to-low lateral osteotomies placed as close as possible to the Maxillary Bone, right above the Nasofacial Groove, as we wish to avoid creating a visible or palpable step deformity in our patients. In our experience, straight, and angled long Piezo inserts are the easiest, fastest, and most precise method to achieve this. We also often prefer to use a hybrid of the push-down/let-down procedures in our dorsal

preservation cases. At the cephalic portion of the bony pyramid we perform an osteotomy (without ostectomy), which is essentially a push-down type of maneuver. At the caudal portion of the nasal bony pyramid at the pyriform aperture (Webster's triangle) we perform a triangular-shaped ostectomy, thus creating a let-down (**Fig. 8**A, B).

We excise Webster's triangle to prevent any potential blockage that may arise when the bone of the pyriform aperture is pushed down and overlaps with the head of the inferior turbinate attachment, which is located immediately posterior to the Webster's triangle (**Fig. 9**). Uncorrected, such an impediment to dorsal lowering could result in an unwanted residual hump, as the bone fragment of the inferior turbinate can potentially block the intended downward movement of the nasal bone. To prevent this from occurring, we recommend that the Webster's triangle be resected when using the preservation technique. This can be easily and accurately achieved with the PEI. A recent computed tomography study has shown improved patency of the nasal area with resection of this region when compared with the traditional push-down procedure.[17] We hypothesize that the reason resection of the Webster's triangle does not lead to internal nasal valve collapse and obstruction is likely owing to the bony support provided by the overlapped bone.

Fig. 9. Relationship between Webster's triangle and the adjacent head of the inferior turbinate, which could be a potential blocking point during pushdown unless the Webster's triangle is resected.

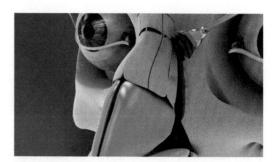

Fig. 10. Transverse osteotomy using the Tastan–Cakir hand saw.

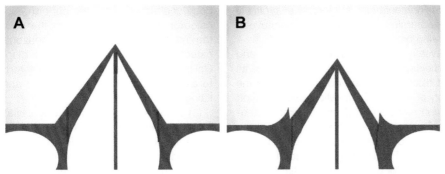

Fig. 11. (A) Sagittal lateral osteotomies using the piezoelectric instrument and (B) push-down maneuver in the straight bony vault.

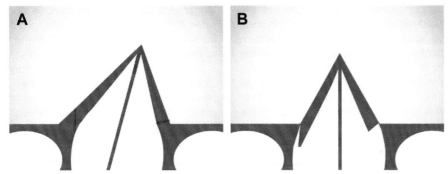

Fig. 12. (A) Asymmetrical lateral osteotomies using the piezoelectric instrument, with (B) pyramid tilting to correct the deviated bony vault.

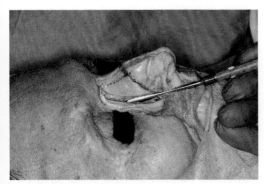

Fig. 13. Elevation of periosteum along the inner surface of the maxillary bone.

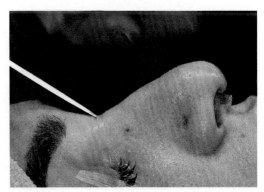

Fig. 14. Percutaneous radix osteotomy in an oblique direction.

In dorsal preservation surgery we typically perform osteotomies and associated maneuvers, in the following order:

(1) Transverse osteotomies: with Group 1 and Group 2 patients, where we preserve the ligaments and do not dissect the nasal dorsum, we use the combination of Tastan–Cakir (Microsaw Medisoft Medical) hand saws and a 2-mm external osteotome. With Group 3 patients, we carry out all the osteotomies including the transverse osteotomies with PEI (**Fig. 10**). The Transverse osteotomy level is highly important for preventing potential step deformities and irregularities in the radix. The best way to determine the transverse osteotomy level is to take the intercanthal area as a guide. If a transverse osteotomy is carried out from a level lower than the radix, such as from the beginning of the hump, the inferior radix portion might cause a step deformity or a low projected radix.

(2) Low-to-low lateral osteotomies: created with the assistance of PEI with long inserts designed by the senior author. There are 2 options for the lateral osteotomies, depending on whether or not the bony vault is deviated. If there is a straight bony pyramid that simply needs lowering, we perform bilateral osteotomies in the sagittal plane. As the two borders of the cut bones are parallel to the sagittal plane (**Fig. 11**A,B), it makes it easier to push down the dorsum without resistance and reduces the risk of residual hump recurrence in the late postoperative period. On the contrary, if the bony vault is crooked, we perform asymmetrical osteotomies (**Fig. 12**A,B). On the short side of the nasal bone we make a horizontal-oblique osteotomy, to minimize posterior displacement. On the longer side, a sagittal osteotomy is used to allow for posterior displacement and pyramid tilting.

(3) Webster's triangle is excised bilaterally, for reasons previously mentioned, in cases where there is no bony vault deviation. However, in crooked nose correction where there is no significant hump reduction needed, Webster triangle excision is asymmetrical. On the longer side of the nasal bone, Webster's triangle is excised completely, whereas on the shorter side of the nasal bone, either a smaller wedge of Webster's triangle is removed or it is left intact and used as a stabilizing stopper/pivot point when tilting the deviated bony pyramid.

(4) The periosteum on the inner surface of the maxillary bone, beginning at the pyriform aperture and continuing cephalically, is elevated on the longer side for the deviated nose and on both sides for the non-deviated nose, to create space for bony descent and to prevent tissue resistance to dorsal lowering (**Fig. 13**).

(5) Finally, radix osteotomy to connect both sides of the transverse osteotomies is made percutaneously in the radix area using a 2-mm osteotome in an oblique direction (**Fig. 14**). Thus the whole dorsum becomes mobile.

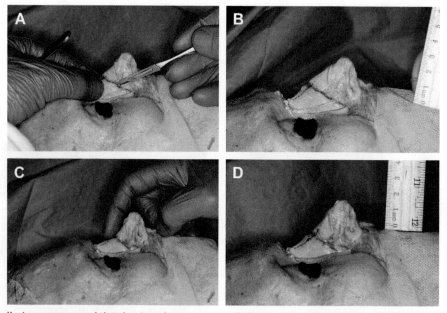

Fig. 15. Ballerina maneuver. (*A*) Releasing the connection between the ULCs and the nasal bones. (*B*) Red line represents the lateral keystone area. Blue line indicates the nasal hump and limit of lateral dissection. (*C, D*) Effective dorsal lowering following lateral keystone area dissection.

In cases of an over-projected radix, following completing transverse osteotomy and lowering of the dorsum, there might be a step deformity caused by high projection of the frontal process and nasal bones. In these cases, we use the Piezo scraper insert for equalizing the bone level. Also, for patients with an over-projected radix, it should be remembered that the sub-SMAS layer in that area might be thicker and there is also the Procerus muscle adding bulk to the radix. In such cases where it is necessary for the bone to be rasped in order to lower the radix, excising the Procerus muscle will further help the skin to settle and hence allow us to create a more defined nasal starting point.

Ancillary Measures: To Control the New Shape of the Nasal Dorsum

It is critically important to understand that the dorsal hump is not a two-dimensional structure.

To achieve the desired dorsal lowering and prevent recurrence of the dorsal hump, there are several ancillary maneuvers that can be used, beyond the previously described septal strip excision and bony base lowering. For example, to change the shape of the dorsal keystone area (DKA) with the high-septal strip approach, the remnant dorsal cartilaginous septum can be scored to further weaken their connection. If a more straight or concave look is desired on the nasal dorsum, the keystone area can be further mobilized by releasing the longitudinal Pyriform Ligament[18]. Rasping the nasal bone's dorsal area, removing the bony cap, and shaving off any prominent ULC shoulders are other additional maneuvers to help the nasal dorsum obtain its new shape.

Ballerina Maneuver (Lateral K Stone Dissection)

Apart from the release at the DKA, it may also be necessary to mobilize the Lateral Keystone Area (LKA) by separating the ULCs from the nasal bone (**Fig. 15A**). The Ballerina maneuver,[19] which involves the release of the LKA side-wall connections, eliminates a potential blocking point causing resistance to nasal dorsal lowering and therefore prevents hump recurrence in the newly shaped nasal dorsum. The extent of Lateral K Stone dissection for each case is determined by the hump height and the desired shape. In **Fig. 15B** one can see that the blue line marks the hump, which correlates with the endpoint for the lateral dissection. Dissection of the LKA, the extent of lateral dissection, and effective dorsal lowering can be seen in **Fig. 15A–D**, respectively.

FIXING THE NEW POSITION OF THE DORSUM

When preserving the dorsum, the final step is to fixate the lowered dorsum into the new position. Once the relationship between the dorsum and the septum is separated, the whole dorsum becomes fully mobile and if it is not fixed to the stable part of the nose, it can move and result in dorsal asymmetry. The method of fixation depends on the preservation septal technique used. Fixation should always occur without any tension.

In Mid Septal/Subdorsal flap techniques it is possible to perform this fixation with septal sutures, suturing the midseptal cartilage end-to-end or overlapping, with transmucosal septal mattress sutures

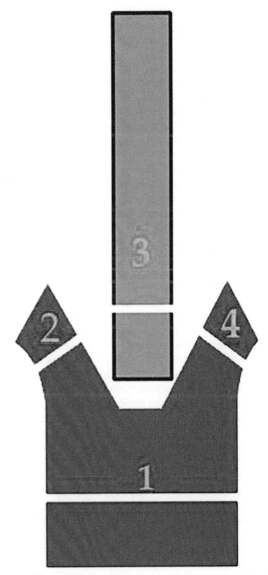

Fig. 16. Anterior nasal spine fixation for low-septal strip single point fixation.

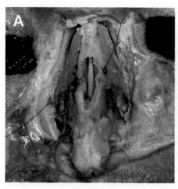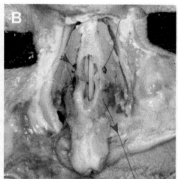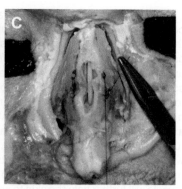

Fig. 17. (A–C) Criss-cross suture for high-septal strip fixation. For illustrative purposes an open roof has been created on this cadaver model, to better show how the crisscross suture traverses through the septum and osseo-cartilaginous vault.

providing further reinforcement. In contrast, in low-septal strip techniques there is a single point of fixation of the freed caudal septum to the anterior nasal spine (ANS). This can be achieved in several different ways, depending on the size and shape of the ANS. Our preferred method is to create a notch with a No. 15 blade on the middle portion of the ANS and then carefully drill a hole from one side to the other with the piezo drill insert through the body of the ANS, followed by second and third holes on either side of the notch. As opposed to standard high-speed spinning drills, the PEI drill device works with vibration, so there is no risk of catching the soft tissue. A 4 to 0 polydiaxonone (PDS) suture can be used to fix the septum to the ANS, passing through the three holes created (**Fig. 16**). In our experience, this method of direct fixation to the ANS bone is the most stable and reliable means of single suture fixation.

High-septal strip techniques require fixation between the osseocartilaginous dorsum and the underlying septum. The sutures can be placed in many different ways but it is important they are not tied too tightly, to prevent middle vault distortion. It is our preference to use the crisscross suture method for fixating the dorsum in open high-septal strip cases. This involves drilling a hole on both sides of the nasal bones using the piezo drill insert. The piezo drill insert can be used to perforate the nasal bones, even when they are mobile, without causing destabilization. Starting from one side and using a 5 to 0 PDS suture, the suture passes obliquely through the nasal bone and dorsal septal cartilage, exiting at the opposite ULC. The suture then loops upwards passing through the contralateral nasal bone drill hole, and courses obliquely again through the septum to exits by passing through ULC on the side of the starting point, and is thus secured. In **Fig. 17**(A–C), an open roof is created on a cadaver (for illustrative purposes only as normally the dorsum is preserved) to show

how the crisscross suture traverses through the septum and osseocartilaginous vault. When the crisscross sutures are completed, the nasal dorsum is fixed to the stable structure underneath—the septal cartilage.

In the Bony Dorsal Preservation technique, the septum is separated from its attachment to the ULCs and at the end of the procedure delivers between the ULCs when the bony-cartilaginous dorsum drops down to its ideal height. After the emerged dorsal septum is trimmed to the level of the descended ULCs, the septum is reconnected to the ULCs using 6.0 PDS, thus fixating the dorsum in the process.

SUMMARY

Preservation rhinoplasty represents a paradigm shift in rhinoplasty philosophy—to preserve structurally sound anatomy and to reshape existing nasal structures into esthetic and functional ideals. Incorporating the open approach to preservation surgery enables greater visualization of the nasal tip and dorsum and provides greater ease of powered instrument access. Furthermore, the addition of the piezoelectric device with rhinoplasty-specific inserts serves to improve the precision and accuracy of osseocartilaginous management and dorsal fixation, thus reducing the risk of bony irregularities and optimizing the surgical outcome.

CLINICS CARE POINTS

- The main determinant of nasal dorsum lowering is not the amount of bone resected but the amount of septal strip removed.

- If there is a need for additional hump reduction, it is possible to incrementally remove more from the dorsal area of the septum.

- Piezo-electric instrument (PEI) preserves the integrity of surrounding soft tissue and membranes and enables more accurate reshaping of the bony dorsum as well as the creation of more delicate and accurate bony work, thus reducing the risk of unwanted fracture lines and irregularities resulting from bony spicules.

- Low-to-low lateral osteotomies can be made in specific planes using the PEI for more precise and controlled "let-down" and "push-down" procedures. If the nose is crooked we perform asymmetrical osteotomies; a horizontal-oblique osteotomy on the short side of the nasal bone and a sagittal osteotomy on the longer side. If there is a straight bony pyramid we perform bilateral osteotomies in the sagittal plane.

- Bilateral Webster's triangle excision can help avoid potential inferior turbinate blockage when performing push-down, without causing compromise to the internal nasal valve.

- Before performing the push-down, elevate the periosteum along the inner surface of the maxillary bone to reduce any resistance to dorsal lowering.

- If necessary, further dorsal lowering may be facilitated with bony cap removal and by performing a limited lateral keystone release (Ballerina maneuver).

- Fixation of the lowered dorsum into its new position should occur without tension. The PEI with the drill insert can be used on the nasal bones and anterior nasal spine to facilitate this process.

DISCLOSURE

Dr A. Goksel developed long piezoelectric osteoplasty inserts with D2 Medical Equipment Company, but does not have any commercial interest or receive any proceeds.

REFERENCES

1. Daniel RK. The preservation rhinoplasty: a new rhinoplasty revolution. Aesthet Surg J 2018;38(2): 228–9.
2. Arancibia-Tagle D, Neves JC, D'Souza A. History of Dorsum Conservative Techniques in Rhinoplasty: The Evolution of a Revived Technique. Facial Plast Surg 2021;37:86–91.
3. Saban Y, Daniel RK 3, Polselli R, et al. Dorsal Preservation: The Push Down Technique Reassessed. Aesthet Surg J 2018;38:117–31.
4. Gerbault O, Daniel RK, Kosins AM. The Role of Piezoelectric Instrumentation in Rhinoplasty Surgery. Aesthet Surg J 2016;36:21–34.
5. Cakir B, Genc B. Esthetic tip surgery with ligament preservation. In: Daniel R, Palhazi P, Saban Y, et al, editors. Preservation rhinoplasty. 3rd Edn. Istanbul: Septum Publishing; 2020. p. 141–66.
6. Goksel A, Saban Y, Tran KN. Biomechanical nasal anatomy applied to open preservation rhinoplasty. Facial Plast Surg 2021;37:12–21.
7. Goran D, Lazovic MD, Daniel Rollin K, et al. MD Rhinoplasty: The Nasal Bones—Anatomy and Analysis. Aesthet Surg J 2015;35(3):255–63.
8. Neves JC. Dissection planes and ligaments. Nice, France: Preservation Rhinoplasty Meeting; 2022.
9. Patel PN, Abdelwahab M, Most SP. Dorsal preservation rhinoplasty: method and outcomes of the modified subdorsal strip method. Facial Plast Surg Clin North Am 2021;29(01):29–37.
10. Neves JC, Arancibia Tagle D, Dewes W, et al. The Segmental Preservation Rhinoplasty: The Split Tetris Concept. Facial Plast Surg 2021;37(1):36–44.
11. Kovacevic M, Johannes AV, Toriumi DM. Subdorsal Z-flap: a modification of the Cottle technique in dorsal preservation rhinoplasty. Curr Opin Otolaryngol Head Neck Surg 2021;29:244–51.
12. Cottle MH. Nasal roof repair and hump removal. AMA Arch Otolaryngol 1954;60(4):408–14.
13. Finnochi V. SPQR technique: Simplified preservation of Quick rhinoplasty. Nice, France: Preservation Rhinoplasty Meeting; 2019.
14. Goksel A. A new concept: structure + preservation. Intensive course: preservation and structural rhinoplasty. Russia: St Petersburg; 2021.
15. Gerbault O, Daniel RK, Palhazi P, et al. Reassessing Surgical Management of the Bony Vault in Rhinoplasty. Aesthet Surg J 2018;38:590–602.
16. Goksel A, Patel PN, Most SP. Piezoelectric Osteotomies in Dorsal Preservation Rhinoplasty. Facial Plast Surg Clin N Am 2021;29:77–84.
17. Abdelwahab MA, Neves CA, Patel PN, et al. Impact of dorsal preservation rhinoplasty versus dorsal hump resection on the internal nasal valve: a quantitative radiological study. Aesthet Plast Surg 2020; 44(3):879–87.
18. Palhazi P, Daniel RK, Kosins AM. The osseocartilaginous vault of the nose: anatomy and surgical observations. Aesthet Surg J 2015;35:242–51.
19. Goksel A. Piezo Assisted Let Down Rhinoplasty. In: Daniel R, Palhazi P, Saban Y, et al, editors. Preservation rhinoplasty. Third Edition. Istanbul: Septum Publishing; 2020. p. 217–42.

My First Twenty Rhinoplasties Using Dorsal Preservation Techniques

Dean M. Toriumi, MD[a,b,*]

KEYWORDS

- Preservation rhinoplasty • Dorsal preservation • Dorsal hump reduction • Profile alignment
- Subdorsal Z- flap • Tetris flap • Foundation techniques • Push down

KEY POINTS

- Dorsal preservation preserves the native dorsal esthetic lines and avoids middle vault reconstruction.
- Surface techniques involve modification of the bony cap and foundation techniques involve bone cuts (push down or let down) with impaction of the bony nasal vault. Subdorsal modification acts to stretch the dorsal hump flat.
- Structure techniques can be used in the nasal tip with dorsal preservation for the upper two-thirds to execute a hybrid structural preservation rhinoplasty.

 Video content accompanies this article at http://www.facialplastic.theclinics.com.

Preservation rhinoplasty is a philosophy of rhinoplasty that is based on the concept of "preserving" as much of the natural anatomy of the nose as possible. The term "preservation rhinoplasty" was coined by Rollin K. Daniel and has become a rather popular movement in recent years.[1] Preservation rhinoplasty can be broken down into 3 different components that include subperichondrial/subperiosteal dissection plane with preservation of the ligamentous structures, maintenance of the alar cartilages with reshaping performed primarily through suturing, and preserving the natural dorsum with possible minor surface modification without creating an "open roof deformity." I believe all these components have merit but the most intriguing to me is the concept of dorsal preservation, which will be referred as "DP" from here moving forward. Many would consider Yves Saban as the person most responsible for the resurgence of

DP in recent years.[2] The history behind DP is quite lengthy dating back to Goodale in 1899 and Lothrop in 1914 and has been accurately chronicled by many.[3] DP fell out of favor with the introduction of reductive techniques and open structure rhinoplasty only to make a strong comeback in recent years.

I have always been bothered by the action of excising a pristine, nicely contoured nasal dorsum to reduce a dorsal hump, only to have to put it back together with spreader grafts and/or spreader flaps. The concept of leaving the nicely contoured nasal dorsum intact and reducing it from below, appeared to be such a sensible approach. Initially, I was intimidated by the concept of manipulating the upper dorsal septum below the hump and making bone cuts to "push down" and flatten the hump. However, I was attracted to the concept and set out to try it.

No conflicts to disclose.
^a Rush University Medical School, Chicago, IL, USA; ^b Private Practice, Toriumi Facial Plastics, 60 East Delaware Place, Suite 1425, Chicago, IL 60611, USA
* Private Practice, Toriumi Facial Plastics, 60 East Delaware Place, Suite 1425, Chicago, IL, 60611
E-mail address: dtoriumi@uic.edu
Twitter: @deantoriumimd (D.M.T.)

Facial Plast Surg Clin N Am 31 (2023) 73–106
https://doi.org/10.1016/j.fsc.2022.08.008
1064-7406/23/© 2022 Elsevier Inc. All rights reserved.

In this article, I will take you through my first 20 DP cases to provide some insight into the nuances of such a dramatic change in my technique for profile alignment. I will focus on the earlier cases where I had problems to provide information to help surgeons potentially prevent issues early on in their own experience.

CASE #1

I searched for the ideal case to be my first attempt at DP. Listening to the experts, it was made clear to me that the ideal candidate would have a V-shaped dorsal hump with a straight-line contour from nasion to rhinion. A less favorable candidate would be a patient with an S-shaped hump who has a pronounced angulation from nasion to kyphion (most prominent point of the dorsal hump; **Fig. 1**).

I also wanted to choose a case where the patient was accepting of a residual dorsal convexity. In June of 2019, a patient presented who wanted a reduction of her dorsal hump but did not want to change her frontal view and desired to keep some of her dorsal convexity. The problem was that she had an S-shaped dorsal hump and a slightly low radix. However, I saw this as an opportunity to do a conservative DP procedure. I performed her case endonasally, and used the Saban style subdorsal high strip technique with rasping of the bony cap and placement of a small radix graft (**Fig. 2**). For the osteotomies, I performed bilateral lateral osteotomies and bilateral transverse osteotomies leaving a hinge (green-stick) at the radix to prevent

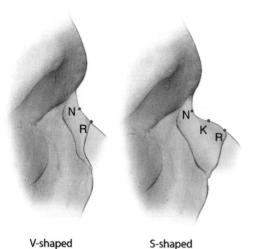

V-shaped   S-shaped

Fig. 1. The V-shaped and S-shaped dorsal humps. (Reprinted with permission from Toriumi DM, Davis RE. Marina Medical Rhinoplasty Cadaver Dissection Course Videos. St. Louis: Quality Medical Publishing; 2021.)

lowering the radix. The lateral osteotomies were performed intranasally and the transverse bone cuts were performed via small lateral wall stab incisions. Before the surgery, I consulted with both Yves Saban and Aaron Kosins who were both very helpful. The surgery went well, and she is happy with her outcome. Her hump is less prominent, and her frontal view is the same by her request. I believe my deficiencies were not extending my subdorsal strip to the W-point where the dorsal septum meets the upper lateral cartilages. This left the supratip too high (see **Fig. 2**C right). I was very conservative with the tip because she did not want it changed so I just placed an endonasal columellar strut. She probably would have benefited from a little more tip projection as well. In this case, I was very conservative to avoid any possible complications.

In retrospect, I thought it went well for my first case and she had no problems postoperatively, and more importantly, she is happy with her outcome. I learned a great deal from this first case. My take home points are as follows. Early on, try to pick cases where the patient would be acceptable of a small residual hump. Many male patients will look good with a small dorsal convexity and may be willing to have a small residual hump. Use an endoscope if you can to better visualize the upper dorsal area where you will be working. One of the more difficult aspects of your execution will be the osteotomies. If you have access to the Piezotome, that will simplify the bone cuts. With my first 20 cases, I did not have access to the Piezotome, so I used 2 mm and 3 mm osteotomes. Starting out it is tricky to make the bilateral lateral, bilateral transverse, and radix osteotomies (**Fig. 3**). In the early cases, it will make it easier if you dissect widely over the nasal dorsum so you can directly visualize the execution of the bone cuts. This wider dissection can result in some increased swelling and bruising so I would recommend a good injection of 1% lidocaine with 1:100,000 epinephrine and also inject tranexamic acid (1000 mg in a 10 mL vial diluted into 60 mL of normal saline) into the tissues around the osteotomy sites.

It is important to avoid placing excessive force on the ethmoid bone while manipulating the bony vault. You can help prevent disruption at the skull base by performing your subdorsal work and releasing the septum from the nasal bones before you make your external bone cuts.[4] This sequence will minimize movement of the bony vault until you have removed the subdorsal strip and extended the subdorsal cut to meet the radix osteotomy. The cartilaginous septum extends close to the radix osteotomy in most patients making the bony cut relatively short.[5] You can avoid a radix step-off by angulating your radix osteotomy, so the

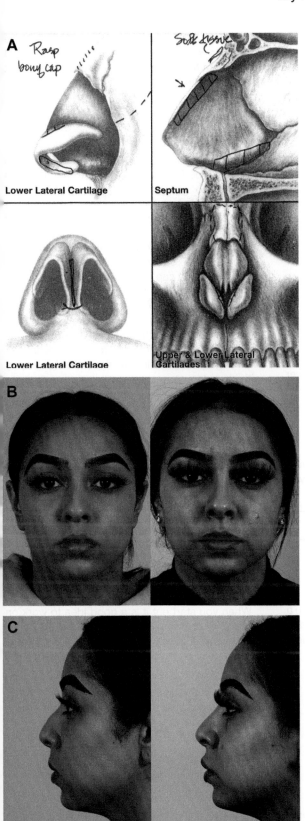

Fig. 2. Case #1. (*A*). Rhinoplasty worksheet showing Saban type subdorsal strip with bilateral lateral osteotomies, bilateral transverse osteotomies, and radix osteotomy. (*B*). Preoperative frontal view (*left*). Three-year postop frontal view (*right*). (*C*). Preoperative lateral view (*left*). Postoperative lateral view (*right*).

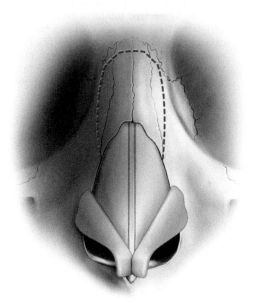

Fig. 3. Connecting lateral, transverse, and radix osteotomies. (Reprinted with permission from Toriumi DM, Davis RE. Marina Medical Rhinoplasty Cadaver Dissection Course Videos. St. Louis: Quality Medical Publishing; 2021.)

upper nasal bone will slide and not drop (**Fig. 4**). This was particularly important in this patient because she already had a low radix. When you are performing your septal work, you must be careful managing the bony septum because it is supporting the position of the bony vault. If you are aggressive and remove a significant amount of the lower bony septum (vomer), this could result in disruption of the ethmoid plate and you may be at higher risk of creating an infantile dorsum due to excessive lowering.

In your early cases, you are more likely to leave a residual dorsal convexity, so it may be a good idea to rasp the bony cap and place a radix graft to help

camouflage any residual dorsal hump. I continue to do this in cases where there is an S-shaped component to the hump and elevation of the radix would improve the profile.

CASE #2

My second DP case was very straightforward. It was a patient with a small V-shaped dorsal hump (**Fig. 5**). I performed this case using an open approach to gain maximal access and to use structure techniques on the nasal tip. I used a Saban style high strip taking out a 2 mm strip of cartilage subdorsally. He had short nasal bones, so I did not perform any osteotomies. I performed a conservative surface modification by slightly rasping his bony cap. I also placed a small soft tissue radix graft. This patient's dorsal hump was small, and I could have just camouflaged it with a radix graft above and a supratip graft below with increasing tip projection. However, I saw this case as an opportunity to use a DP technique. The surgery went well, and the patient is happy with his outcome.

In this case, I realized that using the DP technique is extremely valuable in patients with small dorsal humps. To open the roof of such a patient using a Rubin osteotome or equivalent followed by reconstruction using spreader grafts or spreader flaps seems extreme. It is much more sensible to simply pull the hump down from below, preserving the dorsal esthetic lines and minimizing reconstruction. If his hump was primarily bony, one could have performed a push down by making lateral, transverse, and radix bone cuts or simply perform "surface modifications." His hump was mostly cartilaginous, so it made sense to use a Saban style high strip with slight reduction of the bony cap.

When you start out it is a good idea to work on small dorsal humps (less than 3 mm) with shorter straight nasal bones and a normal radix. Ideally,

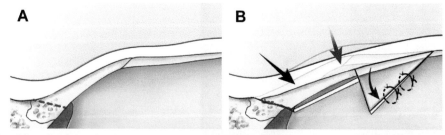

Fig. 4. The obliquely oriented radix osteotomy allows sliding of the bony dorsum. This will avoid an inferior drop and radix step-off. (*A*). Dotted line showing angle of the bone cut. (*B*). After hump reduced showing movement of the bone at the radix. (Reprinted with permission from Toriumi DM, Davis RE. Marina Medical Rhinoplasty Cadaver Dissection Course Videos. St. Louis: Quality Medical Publishing; 2021.)

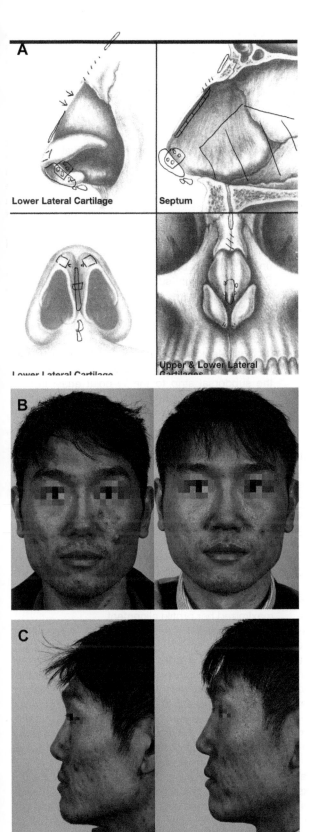

Fig. 5. Case #2. (*A*). Rhinoplasty worksheet showing Saban subdorsal strip, rasping of dorsal cap, radix and supratip graft. (*B*). Preoperative frontal view (*left*). Six-month postoperative frontal view (*right*). (*C*). Preoperative lateral view (*left*). Postoperative lateral view (*right*).

the nose should be relatively narrow in the upper two-thirds of the nose. In this type of patient, a high strip is an easy option and relatively safe. With shorter nasal bones, you may be able to limit most of the work to the cartilaginous middle vault and possibly only have to rasp the caudal aspect of the bony cap. If the nose is straight, you should make sure cartilage and or bone is removed from below the hump so there is no chance for a stump to lodge on one side of the septal strut and deviate the dorsum. The advantage of starting with the high strip is that if you should decide to abandon your attempt at DP you can simply open the middle vault and convert to a structure approach using place spreader grafts or spreader flaps.

CASE #3

This case was more challenging with a larger dorsal hump. I used Miquel Ferreira's spare roof technique type A.[6] I took off the bony cap and exposed the cartilaginous dorsal hump (**Fig. 6**). I performed bilateral lateral osteotomies to narrow her bony vault. Then I performed a Saban style high subdorsal strip and sutured the hump down to the remnant dorsal strut using two 5-0 polydioxanone (PDS) sutures. Critical analysis of the postop result reveals a supratip fullness and a slightly underprojected tip. In this case, I did not extend my subdorsal strip to the W-point, leaving no supratip break. Additionally, my septal extension graft was not as robust as it should be to support her weak tip, and she lost some tip projection postoperatively. Her septal cartilage was very thin and weak. The combination of these issues left her with a less than ideal lateral view and underprojected nasal tip. If her nasal tip was adequately projected, her outcome would have been better.

In overview, my hesitancy to extend my subdorsal strip excision to the W-point has proven to be problematic. My hesitancy to advance the subdorsal cut to the W-point is due to fear of creating a saddle deformity. If she did not want to keep a straight dorsum I probably would have been more aggressive and extended the subdorsal strip to the W-point and also would have taken a larger subdorsal strip. My assessment was that a major issue was the postoperative loss of tip projection due to placement of a smaller caudal septal extension graft.

During this period during coronavirus disease, many patients were frequently wearing masks that can compress the nasal tip. In some patients, I thought the compression of the mask on the tip could also contribute to postoperative loss of tip projection. In either case, robust support of the nasal base with a strong caudal septal extension graft is key to preserving good tip projection postoperatively.

The use of surface modification techniques is very effective and can be used in many patients. Patients with S-shaped humps benefit the most from surface modification such as rasping the bony cap. Reducing the prominence of the curvature of the hump with bony cap removal converts the S-shaped hump to a V-shaped hump that is more readily reduced with the subdorsal work.

CASE #4

The fourth DP case was relatively straightforward. She had a V-shaped dorsal hump and slightly underprojected bulbous nasal tip. I performed a Saban style high subdorsal strip with bilateral lateral osteotomies, bilateral transverse osteotomies, and a radix osteotomy (**Fig. 7**). I used a wide subperiosteal dissection over the dorsum and a Testan Cakir convex transverse radix saw (Marina Medical Inc., Davie, FL) to perform the transverse and radix bone cuts. I did not extend the subdorsal strip to the W-point again in this case. I placed two 5-0 PDS fixation sutures that passed through the dorsal septal strut and the roof of the middle vault. Postoperatively, the patient did well but she lost some of her supratip break over time. The good features of her frontal view were preserved with straightening of her nose. Her dorsal esthetic lines are straighter than preoperatively and her tip is less bulbous.

In retrospect, I could have lowered her dorsum a bit more. I did not extend the subdorsal strip to the W-point. I could have dropped her dorsum a little lower by taking a larger subdorsal strip that extended to the anterior septal angle (W-point). She has a strong chin, and I could have given her a bit more tip projection, which would have maximized her profile alignment.

In these earlier cases, I was acutely aware of the potential for excessive lowering of the supratip resulting in a saddle deformity. These patients did not want a low dorsum or pronounced supratip break. For this reason, I was very conservative when manipulating the supratip area, hence the hesitation to extend the subdorsal cut to the W-point. I do not use fillers in the nose, which eliminated the possibility of filling the supratip if there was a pronounced supratip break.

When starting out, it is advisable to use a wide subperiosteal dissection of the nasal dorsum and perform the bone cuts under direct visualization. If you do not have the piezotome then the Testan Cakir convex transverse radix saw (Marina Medical Inc., Davie, FL) is a very nice instrument to use to

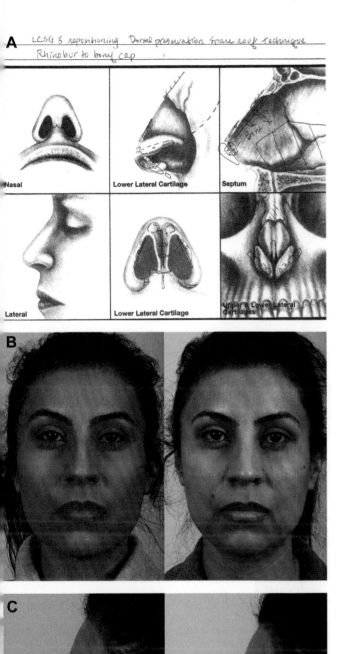

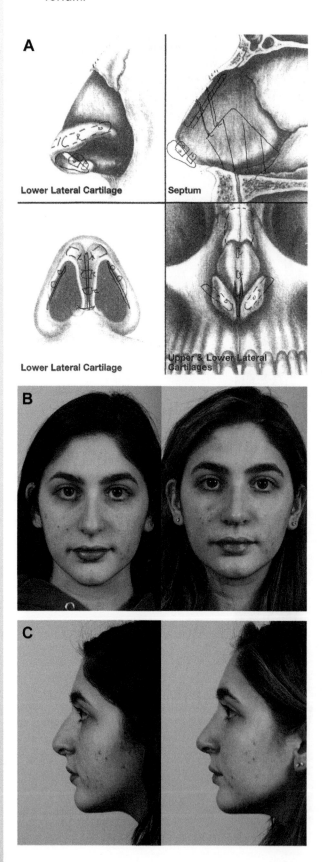

Fig. 7. Case #4. (*A*). Rhinoplasty worksheet showing rasping of bony cap, Saban subdorsal strip, bilateral lateral and transverse osteotomies, and radix osteotomy. (*B*). Preoperative frontal view (*left*). One-year postoperative frontal view (*right*). (*C*). Preoperative lateral view (*left*). Postoperative lateral view (*right*).

perform the radix and transverse bone cuts. The only problem is that this saw tends to create a more vertical radix bone cut that could encourage a drop of the radix area. If the patient already has a low radix, you may want to use a 2 mm osteotome to create an angled green stick radix bone cut to avoid this potential drop (see **Fig. 4**).

CASE #5

In this case, the patient had a V-shaped dorsal hump, deviated nose with a bulbous nasal tip. I used a modified intermediate level strip technique with overlap on the left side of the dorsal remnant to straighten her nose (**Fig. 8**A). The subdorsal cut left more cartilage at the supratip and narrowed as it approached the radix. I used two 5-0 PDS fixation sutures from upper lateral cartilage to remnant dorsal septum. I also performed bilateral lateral osteotomies with bilateral transverse osteotomies and a radix osteotomy. I used a wide subperiosteal dissection to gain access and then used a Testan Cakir convex transverse radix saw (Marina Medical Inc., Davie, FL) to perform the radix and transverse bone cuts.

Postoperatively, the upper dorsum shifted to the midline and the hump was reduced (**Fig. 8**B and 8C). She does not have a supratip break as I did not extend my subdorsal strip to the W-point. I also could have lowered her dorsum a little more and increased her tip projection by another millimeter or two. You can also see that her upper two-thirds is a bit wider postoperatively. This can occur after using DP techniques. That is why it is ideal if the patient has a slightly narrow upper two-thirds to start and a slight widening postoperatively would be desirable.

If you shift the upper two-thirds of the nose to the midline, it is critical to ensure that the lower third of the nose is also in alignment with the nasal bones and midvault. In this case, there is a slight twist of the tip to the right that likely reflects this misalignment. The advantage of the classic Cottle is that you are shifting the entire septum to the midline.[3] At this point, it was becoming apparent that if I wanted to achieve a supratip break, I would have to extend my subdorsal strip to the W-point and provide very good tip support.

Key Shift in Technique

After discussing DP with Milos Kovacevic, I decided to try his modification of the Cottle technique. In his subdorsal Z-flap technique, a subdorsal triangle is incised and the cephalic cut is extended to meet the radix osteotomy (**Fig. 9**). The triangle of cartilage is left attached to the cartilaginous vault (hump) and can be pulled down and caudally to flatten the dorsal hump (Video 1). This is a very powerful maneuver because it acts to flatten the dorsal hump, and more importantly, it leaves a triangular segment of cartilage to easily fixate the dorsum into position. Using the high strip, I was having some difficulty with the fixation. With the subdorsal Z-flap and Carlos Neves's Tetris concept, you are able to suture end to end after making strip excisions if the nose is straight, or overlap opposite a dorsal deviation and fixate to correct the deviated nose.[4,7] I found the subdorsal Z-flap technique to be easy to perform and very effective for correcting the deviated nose.

Up to this point in time, I was using a push down by making bilateral lateral osteotomies and pushing the nasal bones into the piriform aperture. Using the push down, there is the potential for hump recurrence because there are blocking points at Webster's triangle. This area of bone can act to limit the reduction of the dorsal hump and leave a residual hump. At this point, I shifted to performing a "let down," by taking out bone strips bilaterally to remove the blocking points and eliminate the potential push back in the area of Webster's triangle. Initially, I removed the bone strips by making a medial and then more lateral bone cut and removed the intervening strip of bone with a forceps. Eventually, I changed to removing the bone strip with a narrow Cerkes bone rongeur (Marina Medical Inc., Davie, FL).

CASE #6

In this case, I used the subdorsal Z-flap. The patient's nose was deviated to the left, so I overlapped the subdorsal triangle to the right side of the dorsal strut and fixed it into place with a 5-0 PDS suture. I performed a lateral osteotomy on the right and radix and bilateral transverse bone cuts. I also took out a bone strip on the side opposite the deviation (right side) to allow the bony dorsum to tilt back to the right (**Fig. 10**). Postoperatively, she still has a slight deviation of the tip to the left and the slightest dorsal convexity. Some of the asymmetries may be due to her significant facial asymmetries. She has a small disruption in her right dorsal esthetic line. There is a small prominence of her right upper lateral cartilage because it meets the nasal bones. This cartilage "horn" could have been trimmed to improve the dorsal esthetic lines. She is happy with her outcome despite these imperfections. I should have done more work to straighten her inferior septum and could have lowered her dorsum a bit more (**Fig. 11**). I also could have

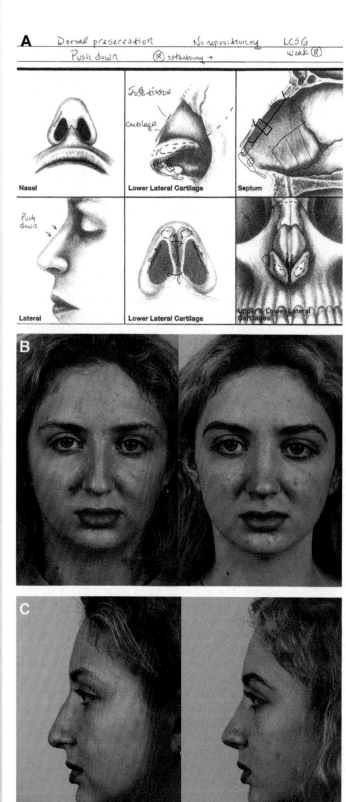

Fig. 8. Case #5. (*A*). Rhinoplasty diagram showing Saban subdorsal strip with rasping of dorsal cap and bilateral lateral, transverse, and radix osteotomy with 2 transdorsal fixation sutures. (*B*). Preoperative frontal view (*left*). One-year postoperative (*right*). (*C*). Preoperative lateral view (*left*). Postoperative (*right*).

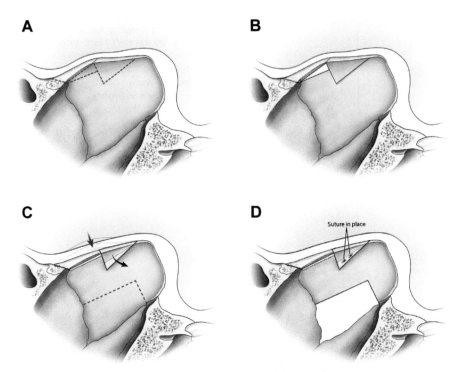

Fig. 9. Subdorsal Z-flap technique of Kovacevic with subdorsal triangular cartilage attachment to undersurface of the dorsal hump with the longer limb aligned with the apex of the dorsal hump. The incision extends under the hump to meet the radix osteotomy. Pulling the triangle caudally and inferiorly stretches and flattens the dorsal convexity. Note the overlap of the triangle on the right to correct a deviation to the left. This technique allows for harvesting septal cartilage for other grafting. This is one of the major advantages with this technique. (*A*). Position of cuts for Z flap and subdorsal work. (*B*). Strip of cartilage removed below the dorsal hump. (*C*). Subdorsal Z flap pulled posterior and caudal. (*D*). Subdorsal Z flap sutured overlapping on the right side of dorsal strut. (Reprinted with permission from Toriumi DM, Davis RE. Marina Medical Rhinoplasty Cadaver Dissection Course Videos. St. Louis: Quality Medical Publishing; 2021.)

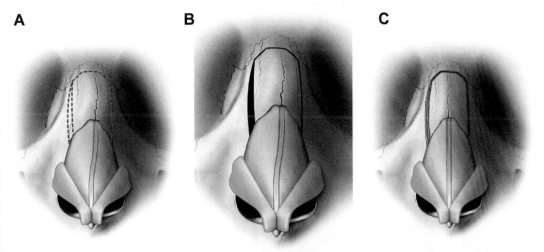

Fig. 10. Unilateral right-sided bone strip removal on the side opposite the deviation to allow the axis deviation to shift back to the midline. (*A*). Planned bone cuts noted in red broken line. (*B*). Bone cuts completed including bone strip removed on side opposite the deviation. (*C*). Bony hump let down and gaps in bone cuts closed. (Reprinted with permission from Toriumi DM, Davis RE. Marina Medical Rhinoplasty Cadaver Dissection Course Videos. St. Louis: Quality Medical Publishing; 2021.)

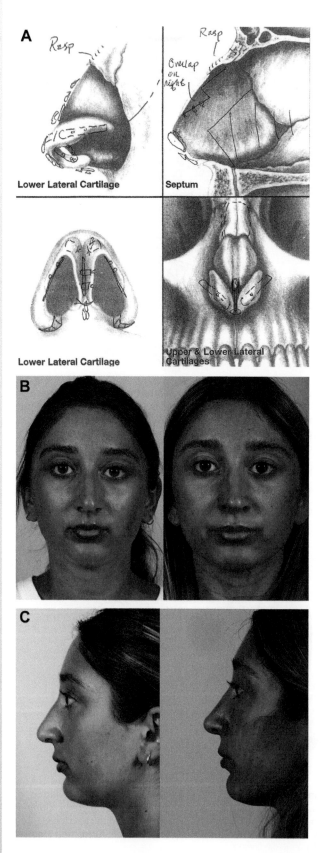

Fig. 11. Case #6. (*A*). Rhinoplasty worksheet showing rasping of dorsal cap, subdorsal Z flap (Kovacevic), left lateral osteotomy, left bone strip excision, bilateral transverse osteotomies, and radix osteotomy. (*B*). Preoperative frontal view (*left*). One-year postoperative frontal view (*right*). (*C*). Preoperative lateral view (*left*). Postoperative (*right*).

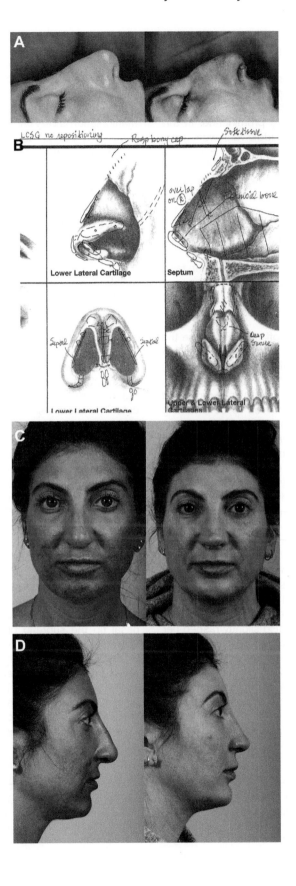

placed a larger nasolabial angle plumping graft to augment her columella/upper lip junction.

This case demonstrates the importance of performing surface modifications to align the dorsal esthetic lines. If one encounters upper lateral cartilage "horns," these prominences can be trimmed with a scalpel to flatten the prominence. In this case, her nasal bones and middle vault were going in different directions. In retrospect, this would have been a great case to use a low strip (Cottle or simplified preservation of quick rhinoplasty [SPQR]) to completely straighten the underlying septum and move the middle vault and tip to the midline.

At this point, I am beginning to get the feel for the operation doing better with the osteotomies and subdorsal work. Up to this point, I have been fairly conservative to avoid complications.

CASE #7

In this case, I was caught off guard because the patient had filler injected into her nose and what appeared to be a relatively straight forward V-shaped hump was transformed into an S-shaped hump once the filler was removed at the time of surgery. This proved to be a turning point where I realized that I could treat larger dorsal humps using DP techniques. I removed the filler to expose the true dorsal contour (**Fig. 12A** left and right). With this case going forward, I changed to using primarily the "let down" taking a bony strip out on both sides of the hump to eliminate Webster's triangle and any bone that could push back on the dorsal hump. I found this very helpful in minimizing hump recurrence. In her case, I resected a bone strip on the left using a Cerkes bone rongeur and transverse and radix osteotomies using the Testan/Cakir saw. Then I performed the subdorsal Z-flap technique to stretch the hump flat and fixated with two 4-0 PDS sutures (**Fig. 12**). I also slightly rasped her bony cap and placed a soft tissue radix graft to camouflage any potential residual dorsal convexity. Postoperatively, the hump is flattened and her tip is projected. I probably could have rotated her more but she was concerned about too much rotation.

In overview, this case was important as I realized I could treat most dorsal humps (V-shaped or S-shaped, deviated), and I also transitioned to using the let down instead of the push down. A key maneuver to consider in S-shaped dorsal humps is to reduce the bony cap by rasping and place a radix graft (if indicated) to help establish a straight dorsal line. This combination of surface manipulation is very important to minimize the likelihood of a residual dorsal hump, particularly early on when you are potentially less "complete" in your execution of the DP techniques.

At this point in my transition, I am treating almost all primaries with DP techniques. I am also modifying my technique as I learn more about the nuances of execution.

CASE #8

This patient was an ideal candidate for a DP technique as she had a V-shaped dorsal hump and ptotic tip with a long nose. I performed a subdorsal Z-flap technique with the subdorsal triangle overlapping on the right side of the dorsal remnant (**Fig. 13**). I widely dissected subperiosteally over the dorsum and used the Testan Cakir convex transverse radix saw (Marina Medical Inc. Davie, FL) to execute the transverse and radix bone cuts. The lateral osteotomies were performed using a 3 mm straight osteotome. Suture fixation of the overlapping Z-flap allowed excellent stretching of the dorsal hump into the flattened position. She had a ptotic tip so I placed a larger caudal septal extension graft and repositioned her cephalically oriented lateral crura with lateral crural strut grafts. Her nose is straight and her hump is corrected postoperatively and her tip is rotated and projected. Her supratip may be a little too pronounced, and I could have placed a more substantial supratip graft to fill it a bit more. Looking back to her preoperative lateral view, one can see that her supratip was already slightly underprojected. Simply by projecting and rotating her nasal tip the supratip break became more pronounced and could have been augmented. She is also a little wider in the middle third, which is also a potential consequence of pulling the middle vault down from below. This can be managed by placing a suture through the upper lateral cartilages to create narrowing.

Her nasal tip was a more significant issue and required repositioning of her cephalically

---

Fig. 12. Case #7. (*A*). Initial intraoperative lateral view showing V-shaped dorsal convexity (*left*). After filler removed an S-shaped dorsal contour is noted (right). (*B*). Rhinoplasty worksheet showing subdorsal Z flap with rotation caudally and inferiorly with overlap on the right to correct the deviation. (*C*). Preoperative frontal view (left). Two-year postoperative frontal view (right). (*D*). Preoperative lateral view (left). Postoperative lateral view (right).

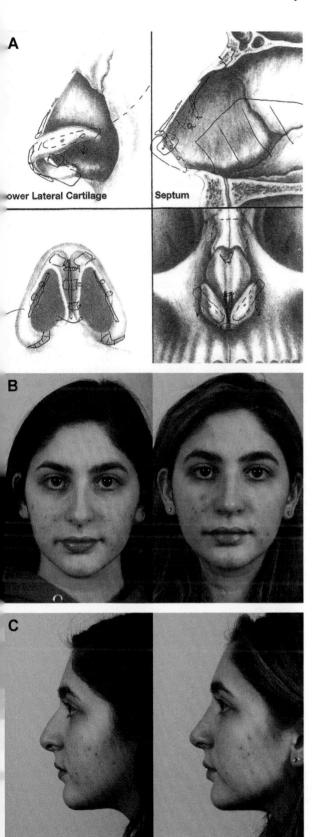

Fig. 13. Case #8. (*A*). Rhinoplasty worksheet showing subdorsal Z flap (Kovacevic) overlapping on the right to straighten the nose. (*B*). Preoperative frontal view (left). One-year postoperative frontal view (right). (*C*). Preoperative lateral view (left). Postoperative lateral view (right).

positioned lateral crura. The caudal septal extension graft was important to set her tip in a more projected and rotated position. With this combination of techniques, I was able to correct the downward orientation of her nostrils to a more appropriate configuration.

At this point, I am comfortable with the DP technique but have not been challenged with a more complex case. My next case was definitely challenging in many ways.

CASE #9

I went into this case convinced that I would perform a subtotal septal reconstruction due to his severe deviation and deviated caudal septum. His caudal septum was off to the right, and he had severe nasal airway obstruction. I consulted with Milos Kovacevic and he recommended a classic Cottle technique, which involves a reverse Z-cut that is made through the entire vertical axis of the cartilaginous septum, pulling the septum forward and fixing it to the nasal spine.[8] In this case, I anticipated that I would have to resect the caudal septum to straighten the deviation. At the time of surgery, I noted the fractured caudal septum, so I released the entire septum from the nasal spine, maxillary crest, ethmoid, and vomer and created a quadrangular cartilage flap (QCF) as described by Finocchi[9] (Video 2). The septal flap was left attached to the undersurface of the middle nasal vault. The QCF was then rotated caudally, and I resected the damaged/fractured caudal septum. To reestablish appropriate length and projection, I placed a large septal extension graft end to end to the rotated QCF to create an "extended Cottle septal rotation-advancement flap" (**Fig. 14**). The caudal septal extension graft

was stabilized end to end using ethmoid bone grafts with holes drilled into it to allow passage of the sutures. This technique can be used for cases with a severe septal deviation or where the caudal septum would otherwise require excision and reconstruction. I also performed bilateral lateral bone strips with an osteotome, transverse and radix osteotomies with a Testan Cakir saw. In this case, I used a septal extension graft and shorter lateral crural strut grafts. I placed septal splints to splint the septum for 2 weeks postoperatively.

Early postop, his bones were slightly off to the right, so I had him do compression exercises on the right side of his nose and his bones have healed in the midline (**Fig. 15**).

There is significant debate as to the effectiveness of postoperative nasal compression exercises. I have been having patients do nasal compressions for years. In this case, I asked the patient to push on the right side of his nose for 60 seconds about 15 times a day. The duration of the compressions depends on the problem encountered. When performing DP there may be some slight shifting that occurs postoperatively. I find the compression exercises to be very helpful in setting the nose in the midline.

Key Observation

This case was very important in my progression as I realized the power of the Cottle technique (inferior strip). It is an intimidating technique as we are all taught to respect the keystone, and with this technique, we are dividing the keystone below the dorsum. The fixation of the QCF to the nasal spine is critical to avoid disruption of the dorsal septal support. In most of these cases, I will make a slight

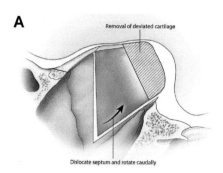
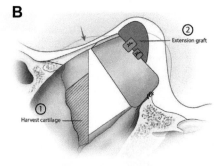

Fig. 14. Extended Cottle septal rotation advancement flap. (*A*). The deviated/fractured segment of the caudal septum is excised to allow reconstruction. Note the placement of the incisions creating a QCF. The crosshatched area represents the area of caudal septal fracture and proposed segment to be removed. (*B*). Note the rotation of the QCF flap caudally to stretch and flatten the dorsal hump with fixation to the nasal spine with two 4-0 PDS sutures. A caudal septal extension graft can be placed end to end and stabilized with slivers of cartilage or ethmoid bone. (*Reprinted with permission from* Toriumi DM, Davis RE. Marina Medical Rhinoplasty Cadaver Dissection Course Videos. St. Louis: Quality Medical Publishing; 2021.)

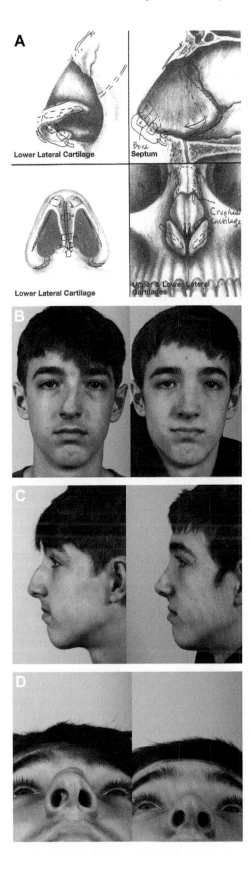

notch in the nasal spine and move it to the midline if needed, then fixate the QCF into the notch, and suture with two 4-0 PDS sutures incorporating surrounding soft tissue and periosteum. Additionally, you can place a notch along the infero-caudal margin of the QCF to prevent cranial displacement of the septal flap.

One of the drawbacks to the Cottle or SPQR technique is there is less potential cartilage to harvest for grafting. If you are planning on performing a good deal of structural grafting (caudal septal extension graft, lateral crural strut grafts), then you may need to harvest ear cartilage. You can harvest some septal cartilage from along the floor and posteriorly, however, typically this is not enough for longer lateral crural strut grafts and a caudal septal extension graft.

The fixation of the QFC to the nasal spine is a critical maneuver. For this reason, there should be no tension on this fixation point; otherwise, there may be a loss of support postoperatively.

CASE 10

At this point, I am very comfortable with DP and feel confident using the subdorsal Z-flap, Saban style high strip, and I have successfully tried the Cottle or SPQR technique.[9] The next case was a perfect case for the subdorsal Z-flap to correct the hump and straighten her nose. She had an axis deviation to the right and a V-shaped dorsal hump. This would be an ideal first case to do DP.

I performed a subdorsal Z-flap overlapping on the left side as well as a bone strip removal on the left and conventional lateral osteotomy on the right to tilt her nose to the midline. I used the Testan-Cakir convex transverse radix saw (Marina Medical Inc., Davie, FL) to perform the radix and transverse bone cuts. I slightly rasped her dorsal cap as well. I placed a septal extension graft and lateral crural strut grafts without repositioning her lateral crura.

At 1 year postoperative, her nose is straight and her dorsal hump was corrected. The amount of supratip break that I left her is subtle and what the patient desired (**Fig. 16**). One could have used a high strip (Saban) or intermediate strip as well. In this case, I did not extend her subdorsal excision to the W-point. The increased tip projection provided an appropriate supratip break.

With the subdorsal Z-flap, I seem to be able to better preserve the preoperative width compared with the high strip. This may be due to the "handle" effect created by the triangular cartilage attached to the undersurface of the middle vault.

In the interest of brevity, I selected 5 more cases out of the next 10 to illustrate due to their unique characteristics. Most of the remaining cases of the 20 are available for viewing online in the supplemental media.

CASE 12

This patient presented with a short, small nose with a dorsal hump. Her middle vault and tip were underprojected (**Fig. 17**). She had a history of prior septoplasty. The plan was to increase her tip projection and align her profile. After opening her nose and exposing her septum, it was evident that a large segment of her septal cartilage was previously harvested. She had enough dorsal septum to perform a subdorsal Z-flap to stretch her hump flat. However, her caudal septum was very weak and needed to be supported. I harvested costal cartilage from an 11 mm incision in her right chest. The rib cartilage was carved into a septal extension graft and other structural grafts.

I incised the subdorsal Z-flap and released the septum from under her nasal bones. I took out a bone strip on the left using a 3 mm osteotome and parallel cuts in the bone. Then I performed a right lateral osteotomy. The radix and transverse bone cuts were performed with a 2 mm osteotome via a small stab incision in the radix area. I overlapped the subdorsal Z-flap on the right side and fixated with a 5-0 PDS suture. This straightened her nose and reduced her dorsal hump.

After increasing her tip projection with a costal cartilage septal extension graft, she was left with a slight saddle deformity. This was anticipated due to the slight saddling effect noted preoperatively. To correct the saddle and stabilize the base of her nose, I performed a "push up" using bilateral spreader grafts that were fixed below her middle vault and sutured to the caudal septal extension graft (Video 3). The subdorsal spreader grafts acted to stabilize her caudal septum and correct the saddle nose deformity.

Postoperatively, the patient has done very well with straightening of her nose, removal of her

Fig. 15. Case #9. (*A*). Rhinoplasty worksheet showing rasping of left leading edge of nasal bone, classic Cottle technique with caudal rotation of the QCF with fixation to the nasal spine, bilateral bone strip excisions, bilateral transverse osteotomies, radix osteotomy, large caudal septal extension graft fixated with ethmoid bone. (*B*). Preoperative frontal view (left). Two-year postoperative frontal view (right). (*C*). Preoperative lateral view (left). Postoperative lateral view (right). (*D*). Preoperative base view (left). Postoperative base view (right).

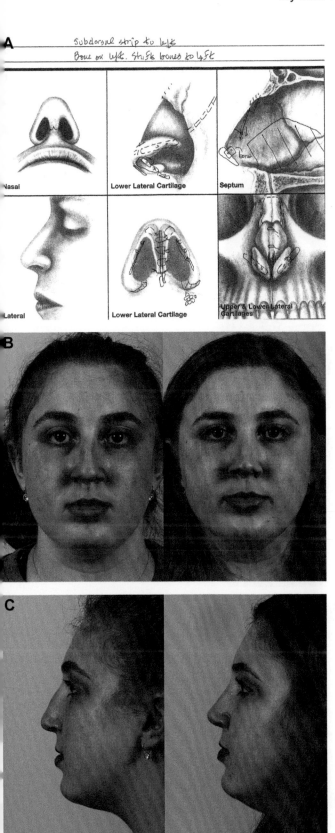

Fig. 16. Case #10. (*A*). Rhinoplasty worksheet showing subdorsal Z-flap overlapped on the left, rasping of the dorsal cap, let down, left-sided bone strip, and lateral osteotomy on the right. (*B*). Preoperative frontal view (left). One-year postoperative frontal view (right). (*C*). Preoperative lateral view (left). Postoperative lateral view (right).

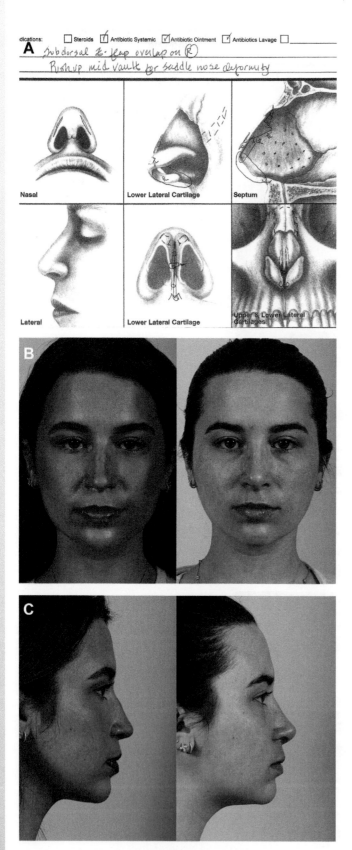

Fig. 17. Case #12. (A). Rhinoplasty work-sheet showing the subdorsal Z-flap to flatten the hump and spreader grafts to "push up" the middle vault and correct the saddle nose deformity. (B). Preoperative frontal view (left). Two-year postoperative frontal view (right). (C). Preoperative lateral view (left). Postoperative lateral view (right).

dorsal hump, and correction of her saddle nose deformity. The concave left upper lateral cartilage was corrected as well. She has excellent nasal airway function, and she is happy with her esthetic outcome. Her nose remains on the smaller side but aligns with what we had imaged preoperatively.

In overview, this case was more complex due to the prior septoplasty. If one decides to perform DP after rhinoplasty with septoplasty, the surgeon should be prepared to harvest costal cartilage and use structure techniques to stabilize the reconstruction. The advantage of using DP in this case was the ability to reestablish her dorsal esthetic lines without reconstructing her middle vault and potentially creating an osseous deformity. The spreader grafts also helped to create a symmetric middle vault.

This case also shows how the middle vault can be "pushed up" to correct the saddle nose deformity. It is critical to use autologous costal cartilage to provide the support needed to preserve proper positioning of the upper lateral cartilages and prevent relapse.

CASE 13

This 15-year-old patient presented with a small dorsal convexity and requested a slightly lower dorsum and correction of her bulbous nasal tip. She also wanted to have her nose straightened. Her primary problem was her wide nose on frontal view.

I decided to perform an intermediate strip (Ishida) septal flap to straighten her nose and lower her dorsum. I chose the intermediate level option to have more purchase to pull her hump down. I overlapped on the left side to straighten her nose. I also did not elevate any of the dorsal nasal skin and left it completely intact. After I performed the overlap and fixation, I noted that her supratip was too low due to the extension to the W-point. This required placement of a supratip graft to avoid excessive lowering of her supratip.

I also performed a bone strip removal on the left and conventional lateral osteotomy on the right as well as the radix and transverse bone cuts. She shifted nicely to the midline. All the bony work was performed from an endonasal site with the radix osteotomy performed from below, and the lateral bone work through lateral subperiosteal tunnels and the transverse osteotomies via small stab incisions along the sidewall of the nose.

Postoperatively, she has done well at 2 years except she has some extra width in her supratip and tip area that fluctuates with swelling (**Fig. 18**). She is taping her supratip at night. I am confident the swelling will continue to subside with time.

This case demonstrates how DP can sometimes create widening of the nose. This is partially due to the compression of the middle vault downward and some splay of the upper lateral cartilages. This can treated with middle vault suturing or slight trimming of the upper lateral cartilages. One can also rasp the shoulders of the nasal bones to create a narrowing effect. Release of the lateral keystone and piriform ligament would likely have helped in this case as well.

This patient was 15 years old when I performed her rhinoplasty. I was always concerned about collapse of the middle vault over time when performing conventional component dorsal hump reduction because this would require reconstructing with spreader grafts or spreader flaps. This area can change dramatically over time with narrowing, asymmetries, and visible irregularities of the nasal bones. With the DP techniques, I am much more confident that she will heal well over her lifetime because the middle vault was not opened and the roof of the bony vault was not manipulated. This is a tremendous advantage of using DP, particularly in the younger patient who will undergo healing over many decades.

CASE 14

This 17-year-old patient presented with a deviated nose and dorsal hump. I performed DP using a subdorsal Z-flap. At this point, I am very comfortable with the subdorsal Z-flap and prefer it over the high strip technique. Because of her deviation to right, I overlapped her subdorsal Z-flap on the left side and sutured fixated with a 4-0 PDS suture. I performed a bone strip on the left and conventional lateral osteotomy on the right. I also performed the radix osteotomy and transverse osteotomies through small stab incisions. I did not raise any of the skin on her nasal dorsum. I also placed lateral crural strut grafts with no repositioning.

At 7 days postoperative when the cast was removed, she had very little edema over her nasal dorsum and her profile was aligned as desired (**Fig. 19**). At 2 years postoperative, she is doing very well with a straight nose and elimination of her dorsal hump. If you compare the 7-day postoperative frontal and lateral views and the 2-year postoperative views, one can see that there is little change during 2 years (see **Fig. 19**). This is likely due to the "no skin elevation" approach to the nasal dorsum. This "no skin dissection" method is particularly useful with V-shaped humps that do not require bony cap modification.

Some people argue that DP is not really "preservation." This is based on the bone cuts and

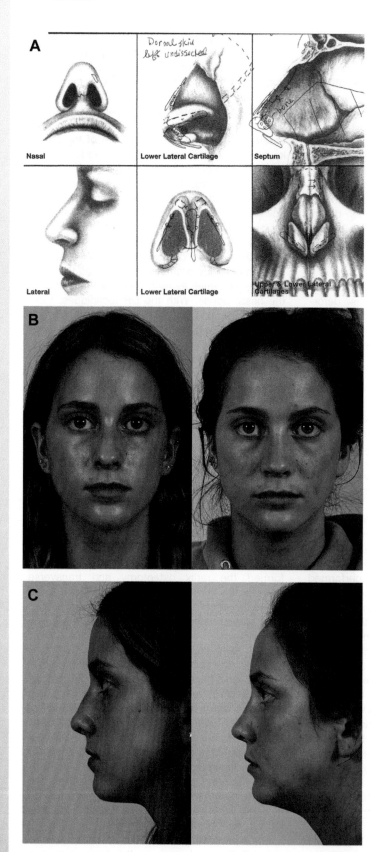

Fig. 18. Case #13. (*A*). Rhinoplasty worksheet showing intermediate level Ishida flap overlapped on the left with bone strip on the left and conventional lateral osteotomy on the right. (*B*). Preoperative frontal view (left). 2 year postoperative frontal view (right). (*C*). Preoperative lateral view (left). Postoperative lateral view (right).

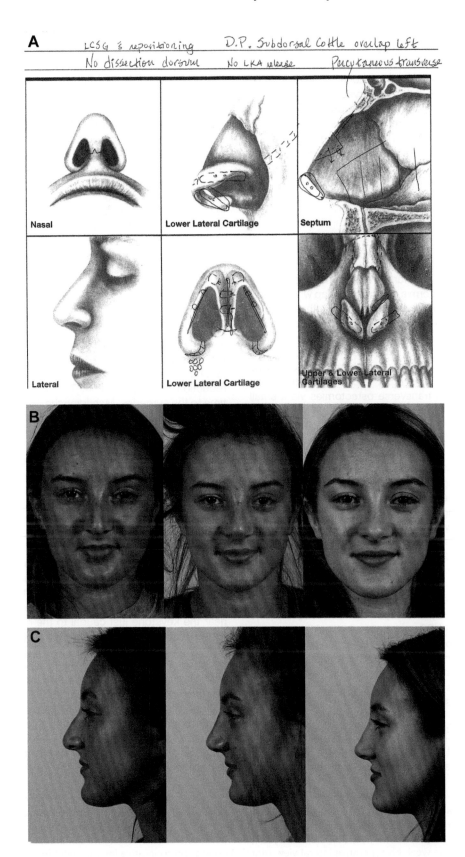

A

LCSG & repositioning   D.P. Subdorsal Cottle overlap left
No dissection dorsum   No LKA release   Percutaneous transverse

Nasal

Lower Lateral Cartilage

Septum

Lateral

Lower Lateral Cartilage

Upper & Lower Lateral Cartilages

B

C

movement of the dorsum as well as the subdorsal work. In this patient, a lot was preserved. With no dorsal skin elevation, all the attachments of skin to bone were preserved. Additionally, the roof of the nasal dorsum was preserved. By performing the work posteriorly under the dorsum and along the maxilla, the entire roof of the dorsum of the nose is "preserved." This is where the "preservation component" of DP affects the outcome by preserving the favorable dorsal esthetic lines and essentially freezing the contours in time.

CASE 15

This patient presented with a severely deviated caudal septum and deviated nose with a dorsal hump. I was planning on performing a Cottle technique/SPQR but on further assessment determined that I could perform a subdorsal Z-flap with a septal extension graft. I used some thin ethmoid bone with holes drilled into it to straighten her caudal septum. I performed a bone strip removal on the left side with a 3 mm osteotome and parallel bone cuts. A conventional lateral osteotomy was performed on the right. I performed the radix bone cut with transverse osteotomies via a small dorsal stab incision over the radix. I overlapped the Z-flap on the left side to shift her to the midline. I performed slight rasping of her bony cap to make it easier to straighten her profile. I used a septal extension graft and lateral crural strut grafts without repositioning for the lower third of her nose. I also fractured her nasal spine to the left to aid in straightening her nasal base.

She did well postoperatively with establishment of a straight nose and elimination of her dorsal hump (**Fig. 20**). I could have placed a larger nasolabial angle plumping graft to improve her columellar upper lip junction. She is very happy with her outcome at 20 months postoperatively.

This case shows that you can effectively combine structure and DP techniques to straighten a very deviated nose and to manage her tip issues. In most all of my primaries, I am combining structure and DP (structural preservation rhinoplasty). I believe this combination provides the surgeon with the absolute strengths of both philosophies.

Key Shift in Technique

At this point in time, I am varying how I dissect the dorsum based on whether I think I will need to perform any surface modifications. In the case where I do not have to reduce the bony cap or place a radix graft, I will leave the dorsal nasal skin intact with no elevation (case 14). In cases where I prefer to rasp the bony cap and/or place a radix graft, I only raise the dorsal nasal skin in the midline and leave the rest of the skin undissected. This approach minimizes dorsal skin elevation but allows access to the bony cap and radix area. I use a narrow rasp to reduce the bony cap, leaving most of the dorsal skin attached. If no bony cap reduction is needed and the skin is left attached, a radix graft can be placed via the small lateral wall stab incisions to avoid the dorsal skin elevation. The radix graft is fixed into position with a 6-0 transcutaneous fixation suture that is clipped when the cast is removed.

CASE 19

This patient presented with a deviated overprojected nose. In the past, I would have to open the middle vault and take down the septum and reconstruct the middle vault to accommodate the reduction in tip projection. This added a lot of time to the surgeries. Managing the overprojecting nose is difficult enough without having to perform spreader grafts and/or spreader flaps to reconstruct the middle vault.

In this case, I deprojected the nasal tip and then reduced the projection of the middle vault and nasal bones using DP. I performed a subdorsal Z-flap and overlapped on the right to straighten her nose. I performed a bone strip removal on the right and conventional lateral osteotomy on the left via intranasal tunnels. The transverse bone cuts were performed via small stab incisions along the lateral wall. In this case, the radix osteotomy was executed by angling the cut into the radix area from below the dorsum. A small dip formed near the keystone just caudal to the nasal bones that I filled with a very thin crushed cartilage graft. I also fractured her nasal spine to the right to shift the base of her columella to the midline.

She has done very well with a straight nose and less projected tip and dorsum (**Fig. 21**). Her thin skin has done well with the DP because there is no deformity of the upper lateral cartilages or bones to contend with.

I believe DP techniques will significantly reduce the complexity of managing the over projected

Fig. 19. Case #14. (*A*). Rhinoplasty diagram showing subdorsal Z-flap overlapped on the left with a bone strip taken out on the left and conventional lateral ostetomy on the right. (*B*). Preoperative frontal view (left). One week postoperative frontal view (middle). Two year postoperative frontal view (right). (*C*). Preoperative lateral view (left). One week postoperative lateral view (right). Two year postoperative lateral view (right).

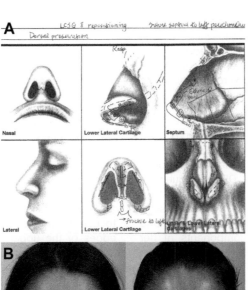

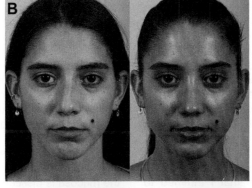

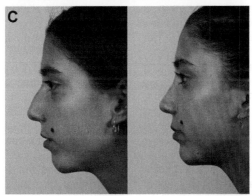

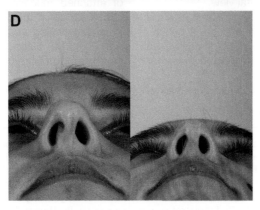

nose as you can avoid disrupting and then reconstructing the middle vault. This allows the surgeon to focus on the complex issues related to deprojecting the nasal tip and not expend time and cartilage on reconstructing an "open roof deformity."

CASE 20

This patient presented with a very overprojected nose and deviation. Whenever we deproject a nose, the middle vault and potentially the bony vault may become redundant. DP techniques are very effective in correcting the overprojecting component of the upper two-thirds of the nose.

In this patient, I deprojected her nasal tip and treated the overprojecting components of her dorsum using a subdorsal Z-flap. She had a high radix so I performed a vertical radix bone cut with a Testan-Cakir convex transverse radix saw to drop her radix. I removed more bone under the bony vault to allow the upper dorsum to drop posteriorly. I took out a bone strip on her left and performed a conventional lateral osteotomy on her right with transverse and the radix osteotomies. With the drop of her radix, there was a slight step off of her frontal bone above the radix osteotomy site. I removed this with an osteotome. There was a prominence of her left upper lateral cartilage (cartilage shoulder) that I trimmed to create symmetry. I used lateral crural release with lateral crural strut grafts and repositioning to decrease her tip projection and stabilize her nasal base.

Postoperatively she did well with straightening of her nose and significant deprojection. Her radix is slightly lower and her dorsal hump is no longer present (Fig. 22). To achieve more dramatic radix reduction, I would have had to perform the radix osteotomy more cranially and also perform a more aggressive subdorsal resection of her ethmoid bone. To be safe, I did not get too aggressive with the bone resection at the radix for fear of widening this area on the frontal view.

These last 2 cases clearly demonstrate how the overprojecting dorsum and middle vault can be corrected using DP techniques. Additionally, the cases further demonstrate the effectiveness for straightening the deviated nose. In my opinion, the ability to straighten the deviated nose is even more important than the hump reduction capability of DP.

SURFACE MODIFICATIONS TO ALLOW DP IN MOST PRIMARY CASES

Several of the subsequent cases presented with asymmetries in the middle vault and required some surface modifications to convert a non-DP case to a DP option. If the middle vault is asymmetric or deformed, surface adjustments can be performed to make the case a candidate for DP. Aaron Kosins was the one who popularized this approach.[3,10] He discusses using the piezotome to burr down the bony cap, trim the prominent edges of the upper lateral cartilages and place spreader grafts when the upper lateral cartilages are deformed. Robotti also talks about dividing the upper lateral cartilages and leaving the septal T, doing subdorsal work and reconstructing.[11] Placement of the spreader grafts with DP can be difficult as you are working in the space where the spreader grafts should be positioned. In order to get around this, I use "submucosal spreader grafts" that are placed into the soft tissue below the junction between the upper lateral cartilage and dorsal septum as performed in case #18[12] (Video 4). If a subdorsal Z-flap technique is used, the mucosa is dissected on the side opposite the spreader graft allowing placement into a submucosal tunnel. In cases where the middle vault needs to widened bilaterally, bilateral grafts may be needed and then spreader grafts are placed in the submucosal tunnels at the junction between the dorsal septum and upper lateral cartilage (Figs. 23 and 24). Then the subdorsal strip excision is performed lower on the septum similar to the modified Ishida septal strip at the intermediate level.[3,13] With the spreader grafts placed up high on the dorsal septum as it meets the upper lateral cartilages, and the septal strip is removed at a lower level just below a couple of millimeter cuff of attached mucosa, the dorsal hump can be stretched down and fixed into proper position. When performing a subdorsal Z-flap, the spreader graft can be placed along the Z-flap on the concave side of the deviation (Fig. 25). It may be necessary to make a vertical releasing incision in the dorsal remnant below the high point of the

---

Fig. 20. Case #15. (*A*). Rhinoplasty diagram showing subdorsal Z-flap with overlap on the left side with bone strip removed on the left and conventional lateral osteotomy on the right. Ethmoid bone was used to straighten the remainder of the caudal part of the septum. The nasal spine was fractured to the left and the caudal septum was resutured into the repositioned spine notch. Lateral crural strut grafts were placed with no repositioning. (*B*). Preoperative frontal view (left). Two-year postoperative frontal view (right). (*C*). Preoperative lateral view (left). Postoperative lateral view (right). (*D*). Preoperative base view (left). Postoperative base view (right).

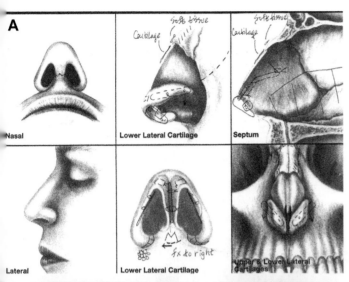

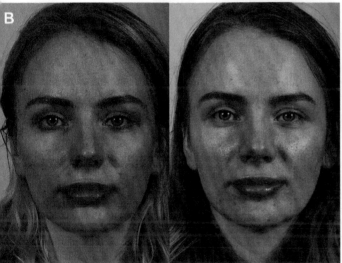

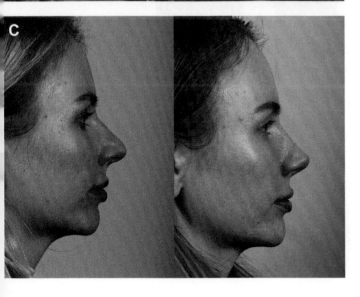

Fig. 21. Case #19. (*A*). Rhinoplasty worksheet for the over projected nose showing subdorsal Z-flap overlapped on the right with bone strip on the right and conventional lateral osteotomy on the left. Nasal spine was fractured to the right. Lateral crural strut grafts with repositioning for the nasal tip. (*B*). Preoperative frontal view (left). A 1.5-year postoperative frontal view (right). (*C*). Preoperative lateral view (left). Postoperative lateral view (right).

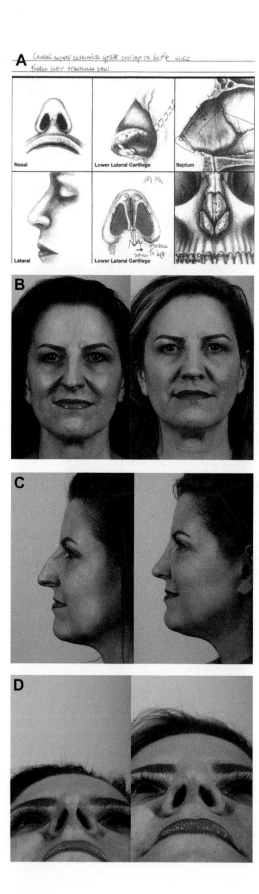

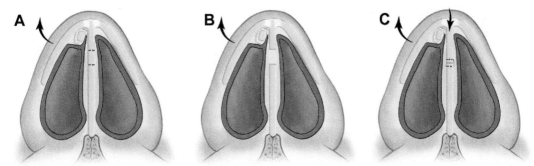

Fig. 23. Submucosal spreader graft. (*A*). Submucosal spreader graft placed into tunnel under the junction between the dorsal septum and upper lateral cartilage. (*B*). Note the lower intermediate level subdorsal strip below the spreader graft tunnels. (*C*). Dorsum flattened. (Reprinted with permission from Toriumi DM, Davis RE. Marina Medical Rhinoplasty Cadaver Dissection Course Videos. St. Louis: Quality Medical Publishing; 2021.)

dorsal hump to allow flexing and flattening of the dorsal hump. Submucosal spreader grafts will also act to tense the upper lateral cartilages to increase lateral wall support and potentially improve nasal function. In some cases, simply by leaving some of the mucosa attached up high on the dorsum on the concave side of the middle vault, the bulk of the mucosa can lateralize the concavity and correct the deformity.

CASES 10 THROUGH 20

In cases 12, 16, 17, and 18, I performed one Ishida intermediate level flap and the remainder were subdorsal Z-flaps. I had no complications, and the esthetic outcomes have been very good. I have 2 patients out of the 20 who have slight deviations of the nose due to correction of the upper two-thirds with inadequate correction of the lower third deviation (Case 6 and Case 7). I also have 1 patient with a prominent bony edge that is not visible but is palpable. There were no cases of saddling or excessive drop of the radix (infantile radix). To date, none of the patients who have undergone DP techniques has undergone revision surgery. The outcomes continue to improve with better profile alignment and fewer cases of residual dorsal convexity. I now also have better control of variations in dorsal height with the option to lower the radix, supratip, and dorsum to create a more curved dorsal line. I am not hesitant to extend my subdorsal incision to the W-point to set proper supratip position and place a small supratip graft if necessary. The intermediate level

tetris flap allows for precise control of the supratip by adjusting the suturing of the tetris flap to the caudal strut.

I have continued to use the structure techniques for the lower third of the nose and nasal tip. In my hands, this involves the use of caudal septal extension grafts for tip support.[12,14,15] For the nasal tip, I use either dome sutures alone or with alar rim grafts, dome sutures with lateral crural strut grafts, or lateral crural repositioning with lateral crural strut grafts.[12–20] On occasion, I will use shield tip grafts in patients with thicker skin.[12] I have been using the structure techniques for the past 33 years with good success. The changes I have decided to make are related to the management of the upper two-thirds of the nose with the incorporation of DP techniques (structural preservation rhinoplasty).[21]

OVERVIEW OF MY EARLY EXPERIENCE TO DATE

It is apparent that there were some issues with the first 6 cases. During this period, I was trying to figure out the techniques and make adjustments based on the anatomy and deformities. The primary purpose of this article is to provide the newcomer to DP some insight into potential issues that could arise and how to prevent these problems. The most important observations that I have made to date are as follows.

1. The blocking points for moving the bony dorsum into position include Webster's triangle, the lateral keystone, and the underlying

Fig. 22. Case #20. (*A*). Rhinoplasty worksheet showing subdorsal Z-flap overlapped on the left with vertical radix osteotomy, bone strip on the left and conventional rhinoplasty on the right. Nasal spine fracture to the right. (*B*). Preoperative frontal view (left). A 1.5-year postoperative frontal view (right). (*C*). Preoperative lateral view (left). Postoperative lateral view (right). (*D*). Preoperative base view (left). Postoperative base view (right).

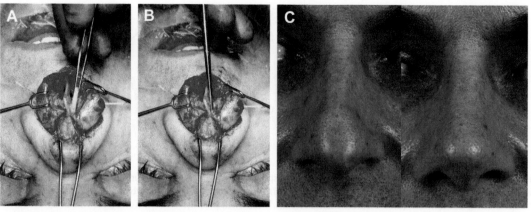

Fig. 24. Submucosal spreader grafts placed in Case #18. (*A*). Tunnels made under the junction between upper dorsal septum and upper lateral cartilages. (*B*). Spreader graft placed into the tunnel under the junction between the septum and the upper lateral cartilage. (*C*). Preoperative close-up frontal view showing narrow lower midvault (left). Two-year postoperative close-up frontal view showing more favorable width of the middle vault with spreader grafts in position (right).

septum. With removal of the subdorsal strip, the septum is no longer blocking. It is important to extend the strip excision under the bony dorsum to the radix osteotomy. In most cases, this is cartilage and can be easily resected. If there is bone under the nasal bones, this will need to be removed with a rongeur, piezotome, or osteotome. If you perform a push down using bilateral lateral osteotomies, bilateral transverse osteotomies, and a radix osteotomy, you will likely need to remove a segment of Webster's triangle. My preference is to take out a bony strip bilaterally in the straight nose and just on the side opposite the deviation in the deviated nose. In some deviated noses, I will take out bone strips bilaterally with a larger strip removed on the side opposite the deviation. I typically will raise a subperiosteal tunnel along the sidewall

of the nose raising the periosteum on the internal and external surfaces of the bone. Then I use a Cerkes bone rongeur (Marina Medical Inc., Davie, FL) to take out the bone strips. The cranial 3 to 4 mm of the lateral bone cut is completed with a 3 mm osteotome to keep a blocking point at the level of the radix to minimize drop of the radix. The bone strip removal caudally removes any blocking points at Webster's triangle.

2. One of the key concepts of DP is the stretching and flattening of the cartilaginous portion of the dorsal hump by pulling the "handle" posteriorly and caudal (**Fig. 26**; Video 5). This can be effectively accomplished using most all of the DP techniques. However, I found that the subdorsal Z-flap, classic Cottle or modified SPQR Cottle rhinoplasty of Finocchi, Tetris of Neves provide the most powerful

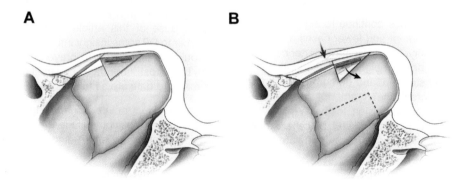

A   **B**

Fig. 25. Submucosal spreader graft with subdorsal Z-flap. (*A*). Note the spreader graft placed under mucosa at junction dorsal Z-flap and upper lateral cartilage. (*B*). Z-flap stretched with spreader graft in position. (Reprinted with permission from Toriumi DM, Davis RE. Marina Medical Rhinoplasty Cadaver Dissection Course Videos. St. Louis: Quality Medical Publishing; 2021.)

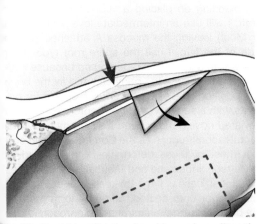

Fig. 26. Stretching flat the dorsal hump by pulling the subdorsal "handle" posteriorly and caudally. This action acts to stretch the hump down at the joint/junction between the bone and cartilage to flatten the hump.

stretching and flattening of the dorsal hump. This is due to the firm connection between the septal stump/triangle/rectangle to the undersurface of the upper lateral cartilages at the dorsal hump. This segment can be easily pulled caudally and posteriorly and fixed into proper position. This segment can be overlapped in the deviated nose as well. Care must be taken as one is placing the fixation sutures because it is easy to pull the suture through the cartilage. To minimize this "cheese wiring," one can leave the septal perichondrium on the upper dorsal septum where the septal flaps (subdorsal Z-flap or Tetris flap) are performed. This adds resistance to "pull through" when applying the fixation sutures (Jose Carlos Neves, personal communication, 2020).

3. One drawback to the action of stretching the hump flat is that the middle vault will tend to slightly widen from its preoperative width. For this reason, noses that start out narrow are ideal because they will likely become a little wider. With borderline wide dorsums, surface maneuvers may be needed to account for the increase in width. One can place a 5-0 PDS suture across the middle vault and bring the upper lateral cartilages in a millimeter or two or shave the upper lateral cartilages laterally to create narrowing. This must be done carefully to avoid creating deformity. For even wider dorsums, segmental spreader flaps can be performed to narrow the wide middle vault.[21]

4. The lateral keystone release (LKA) release or "ballerina maneuver" as described by Goksel

is important particularly in larger dorsal humps because this can act as a blocking point. With smaller dorsal humps, I do not perform LKA release as is discussed by Kosins.[3] I did not perform any LKA releases in the first 20 cases of DP. I routinely use it now with the larger humps and prominent deviations. I think it can help to prevent hump recurrence with larger dorsal humps.

5. When performing DP techniques, you should recognize the potential compartmentalization that occurs with different techniques. When using the classic Cottle or the SPQR Cottle of Finocchi, the entire septum is managed and straightened by releasing and repositioning. With many of the other techniques the upper two-thirds of the nose is managed using the subdorsal maneuvers independent of what is done to the caudal septum and tip. This requires attention to the caudal septum to make sure it is in alignment with the upper two-thirds of the nose to avoid a disjointed outcome (Case #5). I refer to this as "disjointed compartmentalization." In many cases, I am using the overlapping caudal septal extension graft to correct any residual deviations of the lower third of the nose and to prevent disjointed compartmentalization. If the subdorsal Z-flap or Tetris is used but not extended to the W-point, torque can be placed on the caudal septum resulting in deviation or curvature. An overlapping caudal septal extension graft is used to correct these deviations or asymmetries. The side that is overlapped will depend on what is needed to ensure the tip is in the midline.

6. The ability to perform surface modifications of the bony dorsum in the form of bony cap removal, trimming of the shoulders of the upper lateral cartilages and placement of submucosal spreader grafts has been very important in converting questionable candidates for DP to good candidates for DP. Sculpting the bony cap and bony dorsum seems to be a big part of this. In most cases, I make a narrow subperiosteal tunnel and place a narrow rasp to take down a little of the bony cap. Through this same tunnel, you can place a small soft tissue radix graft above the dorsal hump to help camouflage a potential residual hump. Additionally, segmental spreader flaps can be used with the overly wide nasal dorsum.[22]

7. You must become very comfortable performing osteotomies in order to execute DP techniques. If you do not have access to the piezotome, then you will have to become

very efficient at making bone cuts either with wide exposure or with no skin elevation via small stab incisions. My preference is to do the latter in most cases to minimize trauma to the tissues and preserve stability of the bones. If you are inexperienced with osteotomies, your problems with DP will likely be related to these bone cuts (shattered bone, irregular bone cuts, incomplete bone cuts, displaced bone). Fortunately, we have rarely seen these problems in our series.

8. The axis deviation of the nose can be difficult to manage with spreader grafts and spreader flaps. DP techniques allow the axis of the nose to be tilted to the midline with great precision. Treatment of the deviated nose is one of the strengths of the DP techniques. You are able to shift the bony and cartilaginous vault (axis deviations) to the midline with asymmetric bone reduction and overlapping subdorsal segments. I think this is one of the most significant advantages of the DP techniques.

9. The combination of structure and DP (structural preservation rhinoplasty) is a very powerful combination that allows the surgeon to maximally structure the nasal tip and preserve the anatomy of the upper two-thirds of the nose while making adjustments in dorsal alignment.[21] The addition of spreader grafts can turn most primary rhinoplasties into good candidates for DP.

10. Early on, choose patients who have V-shaped dorsal humps and those who would be fine with a slight residual dorsal convexity. If the patient has a lower radix, use a radix graft to camouflage any residual dorsal hump.

11. Follow your patients long term to determine what the true outcome is and make adjustments in technique as needed.

Present Approach

At this point, after performing over 200 cases using DP, I have had the opportunity to use all the published techniques including high strip, intermediate strip (Z-flap, tetris), low strip, and surface techniques (spare roof types A and B). Many of these techniques can be mixed and many are interchangeable. I use the subdorsal Z flap in most V-shaped dorsal humps and mild-to-moderate deviations. Therefore, I use the subdorsal Z flap in the majority of primary rhinoplasties. I use the tetris for larger dorsal humps because it provides a larger subdorsal "handle" to manipulate. I also use the tetris in cases where I must reduce the supratip (tension nose). I can also use a "split tetris" in cases where the bones and

middle vault are going in opposite directions. If I am planning on placing a submucosal spreader graft, I will use an intermediate level strip (Ishida or Most) leaving the mucosa A attached to one side of the flap. I use the spare roof type B for cases with a larger S-shaped hump because it allows me to reduce the bony cap and fix the bone into position. The Cottle/SPQR is reserved for patients with a severely deviated septum or severely deviated nose. I rarely need to perform a subtotal septal reconstruction as the Cottle/SPQR can correct most of these deformities. I have used all these techniques and find them all very effective.

In most cases, I try to keep the dorsal skin attached or undissected, and I perform most of the bone cuts from an intranasal approach (Video 6). I use primarily a 2 mm osteotome and a Cerkes bone rongeur (Marina Medical Inc., Davie, FL). The transverse osteotomies are typically performed via small lateral wall stab incisions. To prevent comminution of the transverse bone cuts, I use a Cerkes hand drill (Marina Medical Inc. Davie, FL) to etch a trough along the intended osteotomy line (Aaron Kosins, personal communication, 2020). Then a 2 mm osteotome can easily punch through the trough in a very controlled manner avoiding comminution.

With the transition to DP, I have actually changed my esthetics of the upper two-thirds of the nose. With conventional Joseph dorsal hump reduction (component hump reduction) and middle vault reconstruction with spreader graft or spreader flaps, I typically left the patient with a slightly overcorrected middle vault (wider). This wider construct was used in anticipation of narrowing that would occur over time due to scar contracture and healing. My conversion to DP has given me the confidence to keep the upper two-thirds of the nose (bones and middle vault) much narrower. I am confident that by not opening and reconstructing the middle vault, I can keep the nasal dorsum and middle vault much narrower as the contracture and healing effect is nullified. This change in esthetics has positively affected patient satisfaction without compromising nasal function. Additionally, because I rarely use spreader grafts, I have more cartilage for the structural grafting in the tip and I rarely go to the ear or rib in primary rhinoplasty cases. These are some of the significant advantages of incorporating DP into my practice.

I have also incorporated a subdorsal cantilever graft to "push up" the dorsum and treat the saddle nose deformity.[23] The subdorsal cantilever graft is also used to elevate the low dorsum in the ethnic rhinoplasty patient.[23] The subdorsal cantilever graft can also be used for elevating and supporting the nasal dorsum in cases of failed attempts at DP (infantile radix, saddle nose deformity). Secondary rhinoplasty patients with a residual dorsal hump and intact dorsal roof are also candidates for DP.

DP has become an integral part of my rhinoplasty armamentarium and has proven to be very reliable with minimal complications.

Final Comments

DP has come back with great popularity. In my assessment, there are distinct reasons for its resurgence. Having the capability to preserve the favorable anatomy of the upper two-thirds of the nose and minimize the need for spreader grafts and spreader flaps is significant. Component reduction of the dorsal hump requires amputating the top of the bony nasal vault and then needing closure of the open roof. This series of maneuvers results in potentially rough bony edges, irregularities, depressions or prominences that may require soft tissue camouflage in the form of temporalis fascia grafts, diced cartilage and fascia grafts, other soft tissue grafts, and so forth. Minimizing this potential site for irregularities is a significant advantage in the management of the dorsal profile. The cases above provide a good overview of one surgeon's early experience with DP. I focus on the teaching points to aid the reader in navigating through their early experience.

The impact on the esthetics of the upper two-thirds of the nose has been a positive change that has improved on patient satisfaction. The incorporation of DP into my practice has proven to be a major advancement in the treatment of primary rhinoplasty patients.

CLINICS CARE POINTS

- V-shaped dorsal humps are ideal for DP.
- S-shaped humps with a low radix are not good candidates for DP.
- Subdorsal Z-flap provides a "handle" to hold the dorsal hump in the reduced position.
- Overlapping Z-flap is ideal for correcting the axis deviation of the nose.
- Let down eliminates the blocking point at Webster's triangle.
- Oblique radix osteotomy helps to avoid radix drop and the "infantile radix."
- Caudal septal extension graft can stabilize and straighten a deviated caudal septum after the dorsal hump is reduced.

SUPPLEMENTARY DATA

Supplementary data related to this article can be found online at https://doi.org/10.1016/j.fsc.2022.08.008.

REFERENCES

1. Daniel RK. The Preservation Rhinoplasty: a new rhinoplasty revolution. Aesth Surg J 2018;38:228–9.
2. Saban Y, Daniel RK, Polselli R, et al. dorsal preservation: the push down technique reassessed. Aesthet Surg J 2018;38(2):117–31.
3. Daniel RK, Palhazi P, Saban Y, et al. Preservation rhinoplasty. 3rd edition. Istanbul, Turkey: Septum Publishing; 2020.
4. Toriumi DM, Kovacevic M. Dorsal preservation rhinoplasty:measures to prevent suboptimal outcomes. Facial Plast Surg Clin North Am 2020. https://doi.org/10.1016/j.fsc.2020.09.009.
5. Daniel RK, Palhazi P. Rhinoplasty: an anatomical and clinical atlas. Heidelberg: Springer; 2018.
6. Ferreira MG, Monteiro D, Reis C, et al. Spare roof technique: a middle third new technique. Facial Plast Surg 2016;32(1):111–6.
7. Neves JC, Arancivia G, Dewes W, et al. The split preservation rhinoplasty: the Vitruvian Man split maneuver. Eur J Plast Surg 2020;43:323–33.
8. Cottle MH, Loring RM. Corrective surgery of the external nasal pyramid and the nasal septum for restoration of nasal physiology. Ill Med J 1946;90:119–31.
9. Finocchi V, Mattioli RG, Daniel RK. Dorsal preservation: a new three level impaction technique with bony cap mosaic osteotomies and no skin dissection. Aesth Surg J 2020.
10. Kosins AM, Daniel RK. Decision making in preservation rhinoplasty: a 100 case series with one year follow up. Aesth Surg J 2020;40:34–48.
11. Robotti E, Chauke-Malinga NY, Leone F. A modified dorsal split preservation technique for nasal humps with minor bony component: a preliminary report. Aesthetic Plast Surg 2019;43:1257–68.
12. Toriumi DM. Lessons learned in thirty years of structure rhinoplasty. Chicago: DMT Solutions; 2019.
13. Ishida LC, Ishida J, Ishida LH, et al. Nasal hump treatment with cartilaginous pushdown and preservation of the bony cap. Aesth Surg J 2020;40(11):1168–78.
14. Toriumi DM. Caudal septal extension graft for correction of the retracted columella. Op Tech Otol Head Neck Surg 1995;6(4):311–8.
15. Byrd HS, Andochick S, Copit S, et al. Septal extension grafts: a method of controlling tip projection shape. Plast Reconstr Surg 1997;100:999–1010.

16. Toriumi DM. New concepts in nasal tip contouring. Arch Facial Plast Surg 2006;8(3):156–85.

17. Rohrich RJ, Raniere J Jr, Ha RY. The alar contour graft: correction and prevention of alar rim deformities in rhinoplasty. Plast Reconstr Surg 2002; 109(7):2495–505.

18. Davis R. Lateral Crural Tensioning for refinement of the wide and underprojected nasal tip rethinking the lateral crural steal. Facial Plast Clin N Am 2015;23(1):23–53.

19. Toriumi DM, Asher SA. Lateral crural repositioning for treatment of cephalic malposition. Fac Plast Cl N Amer 2015;23:55–71.

20. Gunter JP, Friedman RM. Lateral crural strut graft: technique and clinical application in rhinoplasty. Plast Reconst Surg 1997;99(4):943–52.

21. Toriuimi DM, Kovacevic M, Kosins A. Structural preservation rhinoplasty. Plast Reconstr Surg 2022; 149(5):1105–20.

22. Kovacevic M, Riedel F, Göksel A, et al. Options for middle vault and dorsum restoration after hump removal in primary rhinoplasty. Facial Plast Surg 2016;32:374–83.

23. Toriumi DM. Subdorsal Cantilever Graft for Elevating the Dorsum in Ethnic Rhinoplasty. Facial Plast Surg Aesthet Med 2022;24(Number 3):143–59.

"Managing the Severe Septal Deviation Using Dorsal Preservation"

Valerio Finocchi, MD[a], Valentino Vellone, MD, PhD[b],*

KEYWORDS

- Preservation rhinoplasty • Let/push-down technique • Septoplasty • Nasal surface esthetics
- Nasal esthetic polygons • Lateral crus resting angle • Cephalic dome suture

KEY POINTS

- The septum is the most important pillar of the nasal framework; it is mandatory its correction.
- The association of a correct septoplasty and dorsal preservation allows the treatment of the crooked nose and at the same time gives natural results with rapid postoperative recovery.
- The preservation technique is extremely versatile for correcting severe septal deviations.

 Video content accompanies this article at http://www.facialplastic.theclinics.com.

INTRODUCTION

Severe septal deviations are a constant challenge for rhinosurgeonsVideo 1. As the septum is the most important pillar of the nasal framework, deviations of the septum require correction to insure a straight nose. The septum should be on the midline without any tension to ensure a correct healing of the external nasal pyramid.

In certain cases, the association of a correct septoplasty and dorsal preservation allows the treatment of the crooked nose and at the same time gives natural results with rapid postoperative recovery.

The types of dorsal-septal deviation can be various and often the nasal tip is involved.

There are multiple causes of the nasal pyramid deviation and include, in the first instance, trauma, followed by iatrogenic or congenital factors.

All faces present with asymmetry, but most people do not notice this if it is less than 3 to 4 mm.

However, it is very important to show the patient their facial asymmetry before performing the operation as the level of attention to each little detail will increase in the postoperative period.

A careful analysis becomes essential for planning the operation. Each of the anatomical components (triangular cartilages and alars, the septum, the osseous vault, and the pyriform aperture dimensions, the nasal spine, the soft tissues, and the ligament) must be assessed as each can contribute to creating this deformity.

Even though, in structured rhinoplasty, various nasal osteotomy techniques have been described for the correction of osseous nasal deformities, so far surgical strategies have not been described that would be compatible with the dorsal preservation philosophy.

The three main pillars of the dorsum are made up of the nasal bones (in conjunction with the upright branch of the maxillary bone) and the nasal septum. Therefore, the correction of a crooked pyramid must involve the evaluation and, where necessary, management of one or more of these three pillars.

The correction of the septum is essential for surgical success as, in these cases, a major septal deviation is usually present, but the nasal bones are equally important, which are often asymmetrical

[a] Private Practitioner – MySelf Clinic, Roma; [b] Department of Maxillofacial Surgery, "S. Maria" Hospital, Terni, Italy
* Corresponding author. Viale Pietro da Cortona – 00196, Roma
E-mail address: Valentino.vellone@gmail.com

Facial Plast Surg Clin N Am 31 (2023) 107–117
https://doi.org/10.1016/j.fsc.2022.08.009
1064-7406/23/© 2022 Elsevier Inc. All rights reserved.

(Rhinion-pyriform aperture distance can be asymmetric between the two sides) (**Fig. 1**, see **Fig. 4**).

Various techniques are available to correct the septodorsal junction (scoring, crossbar graft, asymmetric spreader graft, spreader flap with asymmetric tension).[1–4]

Although these techniques are relatively minimally invasive and generally produce favorable outcomes, all are based on an L (L-structure) septoplasty. This technique, however, does not take into account the influence of the perpendicular plate of the ethmoid (PPE) on the quadrangular cartilage (QC). Therefore, in the case of high septal deviation, it becomes difficult to correct a septal deviation and the surgeon is forced to use camouflage grafts (only unilateral or double-side spreader grafts from the concave side) or even an extracorporeal septoplasty.[2,3]

On the contrary, for the nasal bones, many osteotomy techniques have been proposed in the literature for the correction of a deviated nose: double lateral osteotomy in the longer nasal wall or, as described by Uygar Levent Demir,[5] a low-to-low osteotomy combined with transversal osteotomy of the root on the long side and a low to high osteotomy on the short side with the addition of a spreader graft from the long side.

Until today, the deviation of the nose seemed to be a criterion of exclusion of the dorsal preservation technique.

In recent years, thanks to the experience gained, Authors have been able to evaluate when this technique was successful or when, on the contrary, it is better to avoid it.

The aim of this article was to underline the versatility of the dorsal preservation technique for the correction of severe septal deviation. In our case studies, 60% of crooked noses present a deviation of the central pillar (osteocartilaginous septum) associated with a deviation of the nasal bones (lateral pillars). The combination of the "Pisa Tower Concept"[6] (**Fig. 2**) with the "swinging door" septoplasty[7] (**Fig. 3**) is introduced. The three dorsal pillars must be trimmed to obtain an asymmetric impaction of the dorsum to reach the midline.

One side of the "tower" appears longer, so the aim is to make the lengths of the two sides equal through an ostectomy of the upright branch of the maxillary from the "longer" side of the nasal pyramid. Once the distances between Rhinion and pyriform aperture have been made bilaterally equal and the septum centered again on the medial line, an asymmetric impaction will be obtained of the osseocartilaginous vault with its complete recentering. On the contrary, the remaining 40% presents only the deviation of the cartilaginous vault (and so only of the central pillar). This group needs septal deformity correction and symmetric impaction.

SURGICAL TECHNIQUE

- The first step consists of a swinging door septoplasty, slightly modified compared with Wright's description.[6] The cartilaginous septum is elevated at the base, in an anteroposterior direction, starting from the anterior maxillary spine to the chondro-vomerine joint and, from there, the QC is completely disarticulated from the PPE up to point E. This enables the QC to lose all influence on the part of the osseous septum because it is totally disengaged. Generally, point E is cephalic with regard to the Rhinion (R) and it may be necessary to also free the R–E segment to completely free the synchondrosis of the keystone to allow a correct mobilization of this joint. Once free, the quadrangular can be considered as a flap that can be shifted both on the sagittal and coronal planes. At this point, the posterior septum can be corrected. Should the quadrangular also be deviated (usually in posttraumatic cases) it is possible to carry out a scoring on the concave side and then, if that is not enough, to graft a multi-perforated portion of PPE with stitches in PDS 5/0.
- The second step consists of the performance of transversel osteotomies using an intranasal

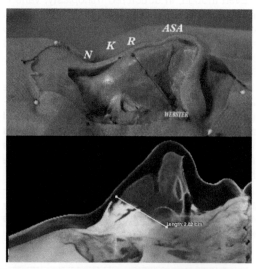

Fig. 1. R-web distance. The distance between Rhinion and the most lateral and caudal portion of Webster's triangle. This distance in a symmetrical nose is bilaterally equal, whereas it is different in some types of crooked nose. ASA, anterior septal angle; K, khipion; N, nasion; R, rhinion.

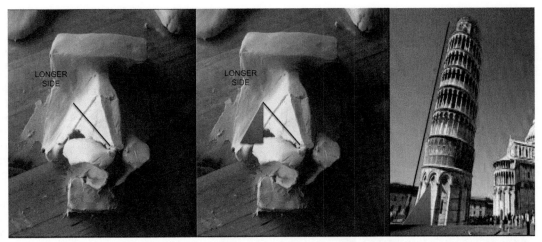

Fig. 2. Deviated and asymmetric nasal bones have been compared with the walls of the famous Tower of Pisa. One side of the "tower" appears longer, so the aim is to make the lengths of the two sides equal through an ostectomy of the upright branch of the maxillary bone from the "longer" side of the nasal pyramid.

approach with a Tastan–Cakir hand saw or through the percutaneous route with a 2-mm osteotome. The osteotomy of the root can vary depending on the case (oblique or sagittal depending on the need or otherwise to modify the height of the root). Now is the time to complete the disarticulation of the nasal pyramid from the cranium by performing either a let-down (LDO = let down operation) or an asymmetric push-down (PDO = push-down operation) or two asymmetrical let downs. A bony wedge is removed from the ascending maxillary process to obtain a greater impaction of one side compared with

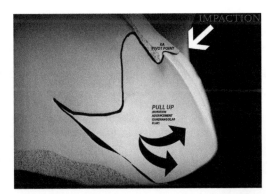

Fig. 3. Swinging door septoplasty. The quadrangular cartilage is detached from the perpendicular plate of the ethmoid and remains attached only to the dorsum by the rhinion up to the anterior septal angle. As it is detached, it can be easily mobilized both on the sagittal plane (thereby being recentered on the median *line*) and the coronal (that is, rotating anteriorly).

the other, based on the preoperative measurements (see **Figs. 1–3**, **Fig. 4**). The normal average distance between Rhinion and pyriform aperture (known as R-web, where web indicates Webster's triangle) in the Caucasian population is 20 to 25 mm (in females) and 25 to 30 mm (in males). The bony wedge to be removed is triangular in shape with caudal base and cephalic vertex. The final goal is to obtain two lateral osseous walls of equal length. Therefore, the osseous tissue that is found beyond the correct distance of the lateral wall must be removed up to the pyriform aperture. If only a straightening of the pyramid is planned, a let-down is performed from the longest side and a contralateral push down (a simple low-to-low osteotomy) from the shortest side, which will make the impaction a pivot point of the pyramid. If, as well as the deviation, it is necessary to reduce the height of the profile, a bilateral but asymmetric let-down will be carried out. The Rongeur is the ideal instrument (especially for those still inexperienced) to perform an osseous resection (**Fig. 5**) of the wedge after a wide internal and external periosteal dissection, but it can also be performed with a protected osteotome (the anterior osteotomy must be performed first to ensure good resistance and stability of the bone during the more basal osteotomy). Following the circumferential mobilization of the dorsum, it may be necessary to correct a slight "rocker deformity" on the side contralateral to the deviation. By removing the osseous wedge, moreover, the narrowing of the inner nasal

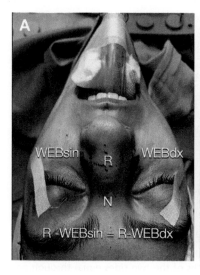
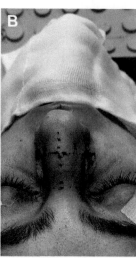

Fig. 4. (*A, B*) Clinical case where it is shown how to regulate the quantity of bone to remove. The R-web distance in Caucasian women should on average be 20 mm. In this case, it is 3.5 cm on the right and 2.5 cm on the left. Therefore, the osseous triangle to remove for the let-down must have a caudal base of 1.5 cm on the right and 0.5 cm on the left.

valve during the nasal impaction is avoided because Webster's triangle will not slip toward the head of the inferior turbinate (**Figs. 6** and **7**). In combination with the swinging door septoplasty, it is possible to correct complex crooked noses without the need for an extracorporeal septoplasty. The dissection of the lateral keystone area (LKA), also called the "Ballerina maneuver", has recently been popularized by Abdulkadir Goksel as an ancillary maneuver in the liberation of the dorsal joint for the purpose of flattening the profile. It is fundamental for us in the realignment of the triangular cartilages beneath the bones when one is longer than the other (**Fig. 8A–C**). The triangular cartilages (ULC) are free to be correctly repositioned with the longer side, which slips internally, whereas the shorter one moves outwards. Furthermore, at the end of the operation, it is necessary to check that the caudal portion of the triangular cartilages does not overlap the scroll area or the respective lateral crus. In that case, a triangle of caudal portion must be resected in

such a way that there is a space between upper lateral cartilage (ULC) and lower lateral cartilage (LLC) where the longitudinal component of the scroll ligament will be repositioned at the end of the operation (Video 1).

As can be seen in the following clinical cases, the association of the Tower of Pisa concept with the swinging door septoplasty enormously facilitates the correction of difficult deviations. Obviously, once recentered, an excessive height of the QC flap will be clear, and its height will therefore be corrected by removing a low strip and refixing the cartilage to the anterior maxillary spine with polydioxanone (PDS) 5/0.

CLINICAL CASES

To simplify these complex cases, the authors have divided them into two groups that will be discussed below.

Type 1. The nasal cavity is not centered, asymmetric osseocartilaginous vault with a septal deviation (Tower of Pisa concept).

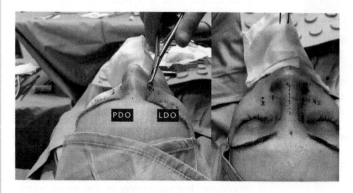

Fig. 5. In this case, in the photo on the left, it is possible to note that the left R-web is correct and therefore the left osteotomy line (PDO) should only act as a pivot for the asymmetry impaction. On the right, however, the R-web distance is 3 cm and therefore an excess of 1 cm. The osseous triangle to remove will have a caudal base of 1 cm. In the photo on the right, it is possible to see that, once the osseous disarticulation has been carried out, the osseocartilaginous vault is realigned.

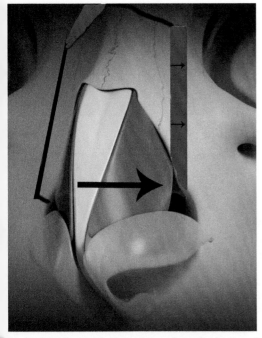

Fig. 6. 3D image. Usually in cases of crooked nose, after performing the disarticulation, a Rocker deformity may be noted along the transverse osteotomy line of the ipsilateral side to the deviation. Therefore, a second external osteotomy may be necessary with a 1 mm osteotome to lower the osseous spur.

It is possible to compare the anatomy of these cases with the Tower of Pisa.

One side of the tower appears longer: to straighten the tower, the longest side must be made equal to the shorter one.

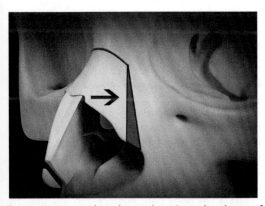

Fig. 7. 3D image that shows the triangular shape of the osseous portion to be removed. In this case, the longest side is on the left and so the axial deviation of the nose is to the right. By detaching the quadrangular cartilage from the PPE, removing the osseous triangle and disarticulating the remaining osseous part, it will be possible to obtain a frontal dorsal realignment.

Removing a wedge of bone (orange triangle), the osseous nasal wall becomes the same length as the contralateral and the nasal "Tower" can be impacted in the right position.

For these cases, the following is performed:

- swinging door septoplasty;
- Tower of Pisa concept. The asymmetric osseous resection of the wedge (LDO) performed on the side of the nasal pyramid
- the treatment of the contralateral osseous wall depends on the quantity of reduction of the nose planned; if minimal, an osteotomy is obligatory from low-to-low without periosteal dissection (this side acts as a pivot and is not impacted); in the case of a greater reduction, a minimal LDO may be necessary as a simple PDO would not be sufficient to allow a reduction of the profile.

Clinical Case 1

Analysis and technique. This patient was operated on by us in live surgery during the National Congress of the Aiceff Society (the Italian Association of Esthetic and Functional Surgery of the Face). Note how it can be seen that the decentered/deviated left nasal cavity presents a longer right nasal bone, a shorter contralateral nasal osseous wall, and a septal deviation with deviated nasal tip. For the dorsum, I used the SPQR V2 technique (therefore without dissection of the dorsal soft tissues) associated with a swinging door septoplasty + osteotomies/ostectomies according to the Tower of Pisa concept + low strip resection and recentering the septum to the anterior maxillary spine + tip in accordance with Cakir. This deformity can be corrected by acting on three pillars, so first the septoplasty, then an asymmetric disarticulation of the nasal pyramid with the following order of maneuvers: external transversal osteotomies + osseous wedge resection on the right + low-to-low osteotomy on the left + osteotomy of the root. Then, on the right, I performed an LDO while, on the opposite side, a PDO. If a greater reduction should be necessary, an LDO on the left side would have been necessary (with a minor resection).

Type 2. The osseous components, the cartilaginous vault/nasal septum complex is deviated and the ULCs present a different cranial-caudal length.

Therefore, it is clear from the analysis that the triangular cartilages (ULC) are positioned asymmetrically under the LKA. Usually, the ULCs are brought ventrally to the nasal bones by around 1 cm. However, in these cases, the ULCs on the

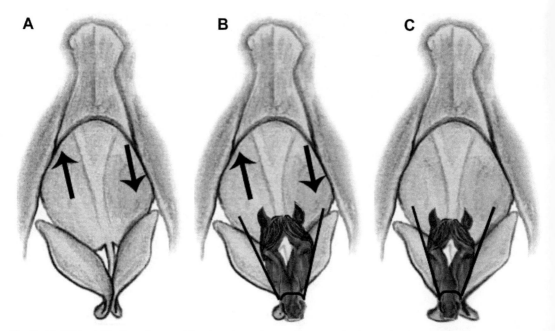

Fig. 8. (A–C) The LKA dissection enables the triangular cartilages to slip beneath the nasal bones and to realign them in their correct position. This movement can be thought of as if the septum were the head of a horse and the triangular cartilages its reins. Once the forces that retain these structures in that position have been released, we will obtain a realignment of the dorsal cartilaginous components.

long side are less extended under the nasal bones compared with the contralateral.

Surgical technique. In these cases, in addition to the osteotomies/ostectomies already described must be associated with the dissection of the LKA as it allows the ULC to be stabilized in the correct position. The aim is to make the UCL slide from the long side cranially and that of the short side caudally. The swinging door septoplasty alone would not allow an optimal recentering of the cartilaginous vault as the triangulars, unless released, would have no way of being repositioned. Conceptually, the septum can be considered as the head of a horse and the ULC as the reins (see **Fig. 8**). After the dissection, the ULCs are free to slide beneath the nasal bones cephalically on the long side and caudally on the short side and the septum is positioned on the median line (**Figs. 9A–F and 10A–E**).

Clinical Case 2

Analysis. The osteocartilaginous vault is deviated with asymmetry of the ULCs. The profile displays a deep root with a slight hump. It can be classified as a V-shaped dorsum.

Surgical technique. The following order of maneuvers was carried out: a swinging door septoplasty + SPQR V1 dissection + LKA dissection + osteotomies/ostectomies with the Tower of Pisa concept (LDO on the left and PDO on the right) + low strip resection and recentering of the septum + tip in accordance with Cakir. The SPQR V1 approach enables the dorsum remodeling, then, once the soft tissues of the dorsum were dissected, I first flattened the bony cap with a rasp, then I performed the LKA dissection. After asymmetrically disarticulating the dorsum and removing the low-septal strip, dorsal recentering is immediately seen. Now the tip, if it does not retract on its own, can be remodeled by performing asymmetric lateral crura steal (**Fig. 11A–E**).

Clinical Case 3

Analysis and technique. All the structural components of the nasal pyramid are deviated to the left, therefore the long side is the left side and the short one is the right (**Fig. 12A–E**). Nasal bones, septum, triangulars, scroll ligament insertion, alar cartilages. Despite this, the patient has a dorsum with good esthetic lines. The dorsum profile is V-shaped and so has a flat bony cap. Authors can say that the hump is practically absent. In my experience, it becomes more complex to realign it with a structural technique than a preservation technique. In my opinion, the preservation philosophy offers a faster and more elegant way out of the realignment. **Fig. 5** is the intraoperative photograph showing how the right ostectomy was set up to ensure that the right

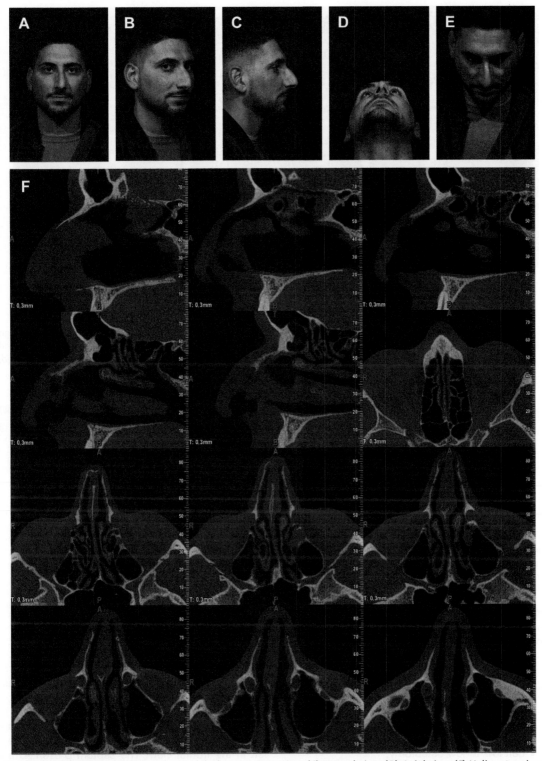

Fig. 9. Pre-Op Patient :(*A*) Frontal view (*B*) Three-quarter view (*C*) Lateral view (*D*) Axial view (*E*) Helicopter view (*F*) Sagittal and Axial pre-op CT.

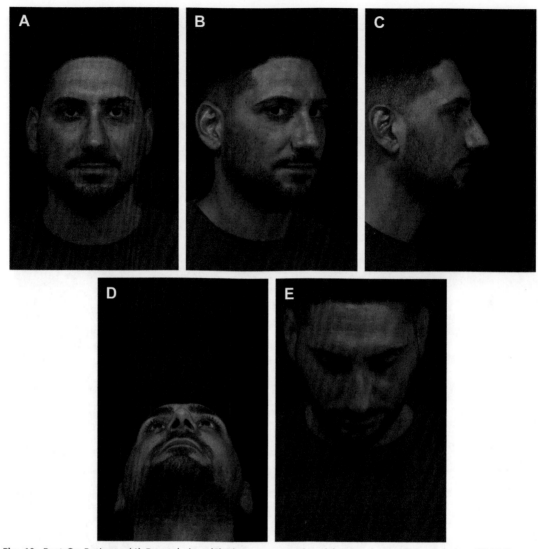

Fig. 10. Post-Op Patient : (*A*) Frontal view (*B*) Three-quarter view (*C*) Lateral view (*D*) Axial view (*E*) Helicopter view. ULCs aree free to slide beneath the nasal bones cephalically on the long side and caudally on the short side and the septum is positioned on the median line

lateral side would become of equal size to the left. In summarizing, the order of the maneuvers was the following:

- Swinging door septoplasty;
- Tip elevation, scroll ligament, and cartilaginous dorsum;
- LKA dissection;
- Transverse osteotomies;
- Right ostectomy;
- Left low-to-low osteotomy;
- Inside–out oblique root osteotomy;
- Low-septal strip resection and fixing QC to the anterior nasal spine;
- Tip recentering with asymmetric lateral crural steal and subsequent asymmetric

medial overlay (more to the right and less to the left);
- Repositioning the scroll ligament in its orthotopic position;
- Closure of mucosa breaks.

COMPLICATIONS

Pre-analysis: patient with an S-shaped dorsum and slight deviation of the nasal pyramid to the left in the frontal view. The septum presented a high septal deviation with PPE on the left. This led to an indirect deviation of the QC.

Operation: a swinging door septoplasty was performed to free the QC–SPQR V1 technique (dorsal elevation) + asymmetric bilateral LDO

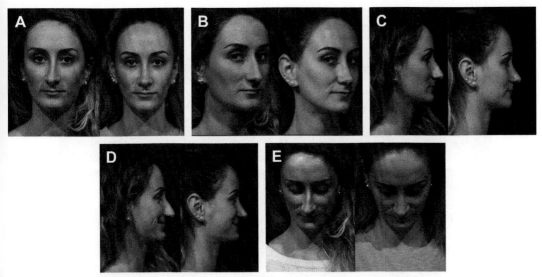

Fig. 11. Pre-Op and Post-Op Patient : (*A*) Frontal view (*B*) Three-quarter view (*C*) Lateral view (*D*) Smiling Lateral view (*E*) Helicopter view.

(with greater removal of bone on the left) + resection of low-septal strip and recentering of the septum on the anterior maxillary spine + remodeling of tip in accordance with Cakir. The elevation of the dorsum enabled the keystone area to be remodeled both with a rasp and by resection of the paraseptal clefts, which were very prominent.

Post-analysis: dorsal esthetic lines not perfectly parallel. At the level of the left lateral side, there is an enlargement of the middle third. The causes of this is due to two possible reasons:

- A septum that has probably not been adequately detached from the PPE and that

therefore continues to exert pressure to the left on the left ULC, which therefore extends slightly to the left.

- The length of the ULC could not be corrected and, therefore, was compressed between the ligament scroll and the osseous nasal dorsum, altering its flattening and causing its curvature.

Even though the level of precision required has risen enormously in recent years due to the fashion for selfies, the patient was satisfied with the work carried out and did not request a correction. But should that have been necessary, what would the authors have done?

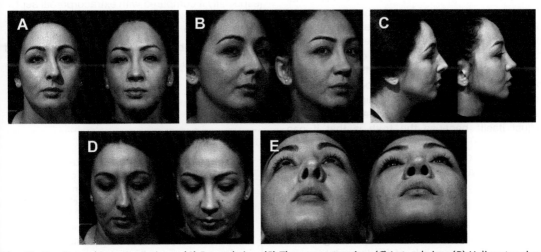

Fig. 12. Pre-Op and Post-Op Patient : (*A*) Frontal view (*B*) Three-quarter view (*C*) Lateral view (*D*) Helicopter view (*E*) Axial view.

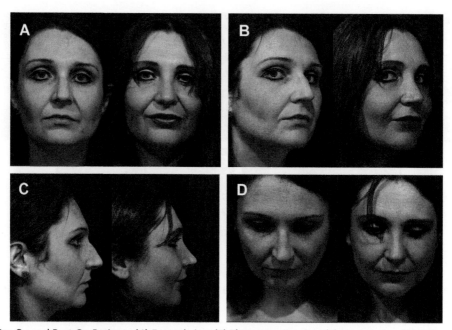

Fig. 13. Pre-Op and Post-Op Patient : (*A*) Frontal view (*B*) Three-quarter view (*C*) Lateral view (*D*) Helicopter view. S-Shaped dorsum and slight deviation of the nasal pyramid to the left in the pre-op.

- First step: a new septoplasty making sure to properly detach the PPE from the QC and checking that the distance from the dorsum to the anterior septal spine was correct. In the case of cartilaginous curvature, removal of a low-septal strip.
- Second step: should the previous maneuver not be successful through an intercartilaginous incision, a caudal portion of triangular cartilage should be removed so that it can be opened up.

This case (**Fig. 13**A–D) makes it clear that there must be great precision in the management of the three dorsal pillars and that nothing must be neglected. The cases have often multifactorial causes that can depend on the combination of many structures. Therefore, at the end of the operation, it is necessary to be maniacal in rechecking and, in the event a slight asymmetry is seen, it must not be assumed that "it will adjust itself" because the truth is that it can only worsen. Therefore, it is necessary to recheck the bony stumps, the septum, the length of the ULCs and review all the steps in reverse order.

SUMMARY

Cases of crooked nose represent a real nightmare for the rhinosurgeon. It is of fundamental importance to analyze the external (photo and palpation) and interior (rhinoscopy and CT cone beam) structures. Once the etiology underlying the deviation is understood, it is possible to apply either structural techniques (which, however, in most cases, require asymmetric grafts) or preservation techniques (that involve acting on dorsal pillars). It is possible to obtain excellent results following both philosophies.

In our experience, the combination of swinging door septoplasty and the Tower of Pisa concept has greatly facilitated things at the technical level as it has enabled us to create a rapid routine (especially if compared with extracorporeal septoplasty), capable of obtaining excellent esthetic and functional results, with a rapid recovery (especially when it is possible to avoid dorsal dissections) and a proper dorsal realignment.

CLINICS CARE POINTS

- It is very important to understand during pre-operative evaluation if the deviation is caused only by the nasal septum or also by the nasal bones as this will change the type of approach of the bones. In the first case, osteotomies/ostectomies are symmetrical, in the second case osteotomies/ostectomies are asymmetrical to push over the whole piramid

- One of the most frequent mistakes during the learning curve of this technique is an inadequate release of the quadrangular cartilage which must necessarily remain connected only between the Rhinion and the anterior septal angle. This allows the quandrangular cartilage to move not only in the choronal plane but also along the sagittal plane. Its anterior rotation has numerous aesthetic and functional effects: it tensions the upper lateral cartilages, contributing to a correct functionality of the internal nasal valve, acts as a septal extension flap, supporting the tip and therefore the external nasal valve.

- When it is difficult to re-centralize the nasal pyramid after having performed the septoplasty and osteotomies/ostectomies, it is necessary to concentrate on the evaluation of the blocking points which can be: the medial canthal tendon, the maxillary bones in case of a narrow piriform aperture, the mesial maxillary periosteum along the fracture lines, the perpendicular plate of the ethmoid and vomer in case of overlapping areas with the quandrangolar cartilage and finally the wrong size of the quadrangular cartilage which can be still to big to fit the space.

DISCLOSURE

The authors have nothing to disclose.

SUPPLEMENTARY DATA

Supplementary data related to this article can be found online at https://doi.org/10.1016/j.fsc.2022.08.009.

REFERENCES

1. Gunter JP, Rohrich RJ. Management of the deviated nose. The importance of septal reconstruction. Clin Plast Surg 1988;15(1):43–55. Available at: http://www.ncbi.nlm.nih.gov/pubmed/3345630.

2. Gubisch W. Extracorporeal septoplasty for the markedly deviated septum. Arch Facial Plast Surg 2005;7(4):218–26.

3. Gubisch W. The extracorporeal septum plasty. Plast Reconstr Surg 1995;95(4):672–82.

4. Gilbert SE. Overlay grafting for lateral nasal wall concavities. Otolaryngol Neck Surg 1998;119(4):385–8.

5. Demir UL. A novel approach to crooked nose in rhinoplasty: asymmetric level osteotomy combined with unilateral spreader graft. J Craniofac Surg 2019;30(5):1512–5.

6. Finocchi V, Vellone V, Ramieri V, et al. Pisa tower concept: a new paradigm in crooked nose treatment. Plast Reconstr Surg 2021;148(1):66–70.

7. Wright WK. Principles of nasal septum reconstruction. Trans Am Acad Ophthalmol Otolaryngol 1969;73(2):252–5. Available at: http://www.ncbi.nlm.nih.gov/pubmed/4890426.

Subdorsal Cantilever Graft
Indications and Technique

Dean M. Toriumi, MD[a,b,*], Milos Kovacevic, MD[c]

KEYWORDS

- Subdorsal cantilever graft • Rhinoplasty • Dorsal preservation • Preservation rhinoplasty
- Augmentation rhinoplasty • Saddle nose deformity • Saddle nose repair
- Asian augmentation rhinoplasty

KEY POINTS

- The SDCG can be used to "push up" the nasal dorsum and middle vault to augment the dorsum.
- The advantage of the SDCG is that the majority of the augmentation is achieved from pushing up the nasal dorsum with smaller soft tissue or small cartilage grafts to provide fine tuning of the dorsal line. This approach decreases the potential for postoperative deformity, warping of the rib graft or graft visibility.
- SDCG is a complex operation that requires significant experience with dorsal preservation and costal cartilage grafting.

 Video content accompanies this article at http://www.facialplastic.theclinics.com.

INTRODUCTION

Dorsal preservation is a rhinoplasty technique that incorporates subdorsal septal manipulation, circumferential bone cuts, and potential surface modification to manage dorsal nasal deformities.[1–3] Preservation of the leading edge of the nasal dorsum allows modification without the need for middle vault reconstruction or camouflage of open roof deformities. The concept of dorsal preservation can be expanded to incorporate repair of other anatomic deformities of the upper two-thirds of the nose.

We have previously described the use of the subdorsal cantilever graft (SDCG) for correction of the saddle nose deformity and also for the elevation of the dorsum in augmentation rhinoplasty.[4,5] The "push up" concept has been previously published by others with the original description as the septal pyramidal adjustment

and repositioning (SPAR) type C by Wilson Dewes in 2013.[6,7] The SDCG differs from these previous descriptions with the use of a robust costal cartilage graft positioned below the bony and cartilaginous dorsum. Additionally, the SDCG has 2 configurations based on the intended effect. The SDCG type A is extended into a notch below the nasal bones and above the bony septum after performing a high strip where the septum is divided from the middle vault and nasal bones. In this case, a space is created below the nasal bones and the SDCG type A is fixed into this space and then extended caudally and fixed to a caudal septal extension or caudal septal replacement graft (**Fig. 1**). The SDCG is then fixed to the nasal bones via a hole that is drilled through the bony nasal vault with a 16-gauge needle or special drill attachment. A 4-0 polydioxanone (PDS) suture is passed through the holes in the bones and then passed through the SDCG more caudally to force

a Department of Otolaryngology-Head & Neck Surgery, Rush University Medical School, Chicago, IL, USA;
b Private Practice, 60 East Delaware Place, Suite 1425, Chicago, IL 60611, USA; c Private Practice, Hamburg, Germany
* Corresponding author. 60 East Delaware Place, Suite 1425, Chicago, IL 60611.
E-mail address: deantoriumi@toriumimd.com
Twitter: @deantoriumimd (D.M.T.)

Facial Plast Surg Clin N Am 31 (2023) 119–129
https://doi.org/10.1016/j.fsc.2022.08.006
1064-7406/23/© 2022 Elsevier Inc. All rights reserved.

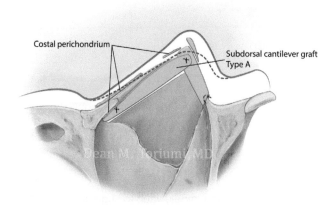

Costal perichondrium

Subdorsal cantilever graft
Type A

Fig. 1. SDCG type A with extension of the graft into a gap created between the undersurface of the nasal bones and the ethmoid bone. Note the graft does not extend through the radix osteotomy site. The graft is fixed caudally to the caudal septal extension graft. (Used from the library of Dean M. Toriumi with permission. Figure is copyrighted by the author, Dean M. Toriumi ©)

the graft cranially. This configuration of the SDCG is used for repair of the saddle nose deformity and for correction of the severely deviated nose.[4]

The SDCG type B is used in cases where the radix position needs to be elevated and/or shifted (**Fig. 2**). This is used primarily for major dorsal augmentation and in cases of ethnic augmentation rhinoplasty.[5] The SDCG type B can also be used when there is complete loss of subdorsal septal support during a dorsal preservation procedure. It is possible that with execution of the subdorsal septal work and bone work, the supportive nature of the nasal septum is compromised. In these cases, there is risk that the nasal dorsum could "collapse." The SDCG type B can be used as a "bail out" for this difficult scenario.

Autologous costal cartilage is recommended for all SDCG's and ideally the cartilage should be dense or partially calcified. The harvested rib should be carved in an axial plane (from anterior to posterior), taking about 50% of the height of the harvested segment for the SDCG (180° of the native edge). The native perichondrium should be left on at least one edge of the harvested cartilage to aid in fixation and to help stabilize the graft. If the rib segment is narrow, then the entire segment can be used as the SDCG. This will maximize strength of the graft and also will minimize the chance of warping.[5] If soft costal cartilage is encountered, then a costochondral rib segment should be harvested to provide the necessary rigidity to support the dorsum and middle vault. If strong costal cartilage segments are not available, then other treatment options should be considered.

SUBDORSAL CANTILEVER GRAFT TYPE A FOR REPAIR OF THE SADDLE NOSE DEFORMITY

In most saddle nose deformities, there is loss of cartilaginous septal support under the middle

nasal vault resulting in the loss of projection with the resultant saddling of the middle nasal vault. To repair the saddle nose deformity, costal cartilage is harvested. We typically harvest the sixth or seventh rib through an inframammary incision. The SDCG is carved into a graft that is typically 3.5 to 4 cm in length and 7 to 10 mm in depth. The width varies depending on the desired width of the nasal dorsum. If a narrower dorsum is desired, then the graft should come to a peak. A groove can also be carved into the leading edge to accommodate any remnant dorsal septum left on the undersurface of the nasal dorsum (**Fig. 3**). *The SDCG should have a prominence where the graft sits under the middle vault to insure adequate elevation of the middle third of the nose.* In order to allow the middle vault to elevate to the desired level, the upper lateral cartilages and caudal nasal bones must be divided from the underlying septum. To accomplish this, a high septal cut is performed using a straight scissors or 11 blade where the septum is divided from the bony and cartilaginous vault. The subdorsal cut is extended under the nasal bones. A gap is created under the nasal bones by removing a strip of cartilage and/or bone. This space is created to accommodate the upper aspect of the SDCG type A. A lateral osteotomy is performed bilaterally with wide elevation of the periosteum over the maxilla to allow elevation. With longer nasal bones, it may be necessary to perform transverse bone cuts and a green stick radix bone cut as well (**Fig. 4**). If the nasal bones are short then no bone cuts may be necessary. Then the upper lateral cartilage must be released from the piriform aperture to allow elevation of the middle nasal vault (**Fig. 5**). This can be accomplished by performing a full lateral keystone release and division of the piriform ligament (Video 1). A wide dissection of the periosteum

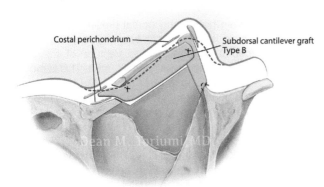

Fig. 2. SDCG type B with cranial extension of the graft extending though the radix osteotomy site and sitting on top of the frontal bone. The graft acts to raise the dorsum and radix. The upper end of the graft is camouflaged with perichondrium or other soft tissues. (Used from the library of Dean M. Toriumi with permission. Figure is copyrighted by the author, Dean M. Toriumi ©)

on the inner surface of the piriform aperture is important as well. In some cases where the mucosa is scarred, a release of the mucosa may be necessary.

In the classic saddle nose deformity, the patient may have a dorsal hump in addition to the low saddled middle vault. To create a straight dorsum, it may be necessary to reduce the bony cap and raise the saddled middle vault to fully correct the profile alignment (**Fig. 6**). In some cases, the dorsal hump can be reduced using a let down with surface techniques. In many cases, some refinement

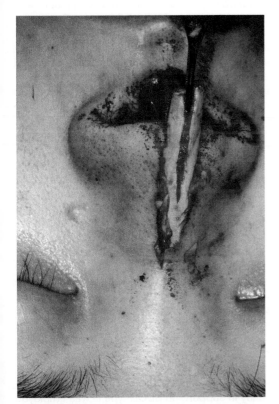

Fig. 3. The SDCG can have a groove carved in the upper surface to accommodate the stump of septum on the undersurface of the bony and cartilaginous dorsum. If there is no stump then the groove is not needed.

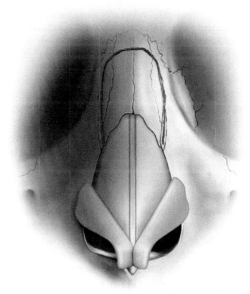

Fig. 4. The bony and cartilaginous vaults are freed up by performing bilateral lateral osteotomies, bilateral transverse osteotomies, and a radix osteotomy. (Reprinted with permission from Toriumi DM, Davis RE. Marina Medical Rhinoplasty Cadaver Dissection Course Videos. St. Louis: Quality Medical Publishing; 2021)

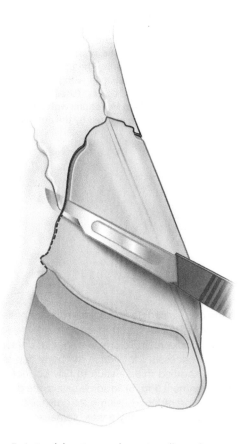

Fig. 5. Lateral keystone release to allow the upper lateral cartilages to be pushed up. If full release is not accomplished, then relapse is more likely. (Reprinted with permission from Toriumi DM, Davis RE. Marina Medical Rhinoplasty Cadaver Dissection Course videos. St. Louis: Quality Medical Publishing; 2021)

of the profile may be necessary by placing some small soft cartilage or soft tissue grafts (perichondrium) to create the final profile contour.

In some patients where the nasal tip is projected, a saddling effect can be noted due to the increase in tip projection in relation to the dorsum. This is a common finding in patients who suffered nasal trauma or have an inherently low dorsum. In these cases, the middle vault can be raised to complement the increase in nasal tip projection and create a balanced profile. The SDCG type A can be used to raise the middle vault after release of the lateral keystone area and piriform ligament (**Fig. 7**). In many of these patients, the saddling is hidden due to thicker skin or the supratip skin draping from the tip to the bony dorsum. Once the middle vault is dissected one can note the severe deficiency in middle vault projection. This deficiency can be corrected with the SDCG type A.

SUBDORSAL CANTILEVER GRAFT FOR SALVAGE OF FAILED DORSAL PRESERVATION OPERATION

When performing dorsal preservation techniques, there is the possibility of loss of the underlying septal support due to fracture of the ethmoid, vomer, and dorsal septal L-strut. This is most likely after the surgeon has completed the release from the bony dorsum and middle vault and septal cartilage is harvested posteriorly and inferiorly. This can also occur during execution of the low strip (Cottle, Septal pyramidal adjustment and repositioning [SPQR] of Finocchi or SPAR B). If the quadrangular cartilage flap (QCF) is weak, too short, damaged, and cannot be adequately fixed to the nasal spine, the nasal bones and middle vault could lose support creating deformity. If this should occur, the surgeon can resort to structure techniques to reestablish dorsal septal support. The problem may be the lack of a stable nasal bone structure or bony septal support to fix spreader grafts or a dorsal graft to reestablish an L-strut structure.

As a potential "bailout" for loss of septal support while performing dorsal preservation, the SDCG type B can be used to create a new dorsal L-strut support structure. The SDCG type B can be advanced through the radix osteotomy site and fixed to the remnant frontal bone at the radix area and then fixed caudally to a caudal septal replacement graft. In some cases, a transcutaneous threaded Kirschner wire can be used to fixate the SDCG type B to the frontal bone. The K-wire can be removed on postoperative day 7. Using the SDCG type B, the entire bony dorsum and middle vault can be stabilized from below. As with the saddle nose push up, release at the lateral keystone and release of the piriform ligament may be needed. Wide dissection around the osteotomy sites may also be necessary. This is an example of how structure and dorsal preservation can be combined in a hybrid approach.

In patients with severe septal deformities, SDCG type B grafts can be helpful if the QCF flap is too short or damaged to adequately reach the nasal spine while performing a Cottle/SPQR maneuver. As shown in **Fig. 8**, a patient with a severely deviated nose and severe septal deformity was treated with a Cottle/SPQR but the deformed QCF was found to be too short and damaged to adequately reach the nasal spine. In this case, there was loss of bony support from the septum as well. To correct the deficiency in support, an SDCG type B was employed using the patient's costal cartilage (see **Fig. 8**). During the procedure, it was evident that the QCF would not support the bony dorsum and middle vault (Video 2). The SDCG type B was advanced through

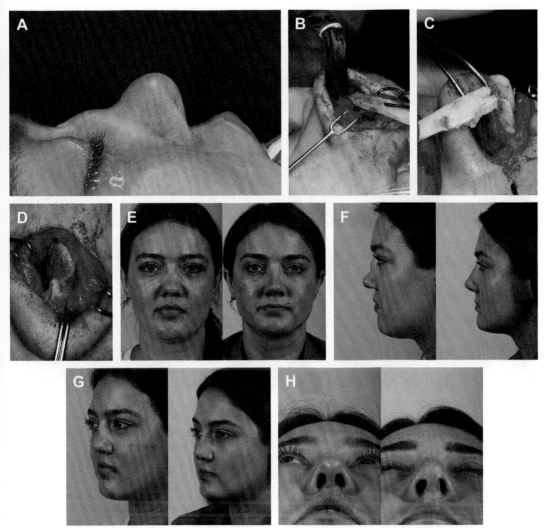

Fig. 6. Patient with a classic saddle nose deformity. (*A*) Intraoperative lateral view showing saddle nose deformity. (*B*) SDCG carved to fit under the bony and cartilaginous vaults. (*C*) The caudal end of the graft is notched to fix to the caudal septal extension graft. (*D*) The SDCG is fixed to the caudal septal extension graft. (*E*) Preoperative frontal view (left). One-year postoperative frontal view (right). (*F*) Preoperative lateral view (left). Postoperative lateral view (right). (*G*) Preoperative oblique view (left). Postoperative lateral view (right). (*H*) Preoperative base view (left). Postoperative base view (right).

the radix osteotomy site and fixed to the nasal bones and fixed inferiorly to a caudal septal replacement graft. The patient has done well with good dorsal septal support and straightening of his nose. This patient also demonstrates how the SDCG can be used to straighten a severely deviated nose by releasing all the septal attachments and placing an SDCG that is either in the midline or off center to straighten a deviated nose.

With a severe middle vault deformity, the SDCG can be shifted to the side opposite the subdorsal stump under the middle vault to shift the middle vault to the midline. In cases with an S-shaped deviation, a custom-designed SDCG with a slight opposing curvature can be used to straighten these complex deviations. The SDCG type B provides the surgeon with complete control of the position and contour of the upper two-thirds of the nose.

SUBDORSAL CANTILEVER GRAFT FOR RAISING THE NASAL DORSUM

The SDCG can also be used to raise the nasal dorsum in patients who desire dorsal augmentation. If the dorsum is elevated but the radix is left in the same position, then an SDCG type A is used. In this case, the middle vault and caudal nasal bones are released from the septum (high strip) and can be elevated to accommodate increases in nasal tip projection.

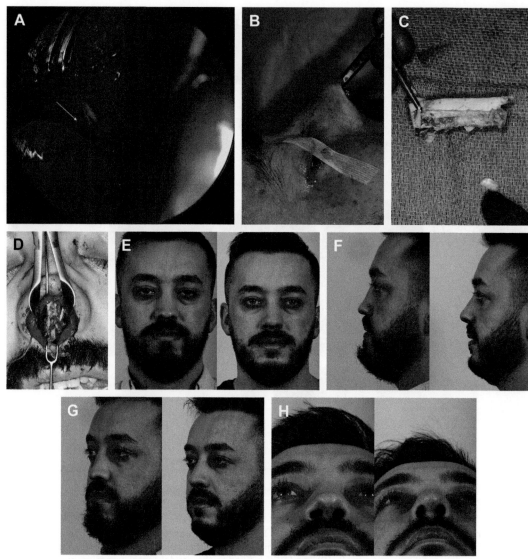

Fig. 7. Patient with a low dorsum and underprojected tip. (*A*) After the release of the septum from the bony and cartilaginous vaults. Yellow arrow points to the gap between the septum and cartilaginous vault. (*B*) After completion of bone cuts a 2 mm osteotome is used to elevate the bony and cartilaginous vaults. (*C*) SDCG with notch that will set into the radix osteotomy site. (*D*) SDCG is fixed to the caudal septal extension graft. (*E*) Preoperative frontal view (left). Eight-month postoperative frontal view showing excellent narrowing of the bony vault (right). (*F*) Preoperative lateral view (left). Postoperative lateral view (right). (*G*) Preoperative oblique view (left). Postoperative oblique view (right). (*H*) Preoperative base view (left). Postoperative base view (right).

Many Asian patients desire to have their tip projected with minimal elevation of their radix. To accomplish this, a large caudal septal extension graft is used to stabilize the base of the nose and increase tip projection. This is frequently combined with a shield tip graft and lateral crural grafts or articulated rim grafts.[8] The middle vault and caudal nasal bones can be elevated using the SDCG type A to complement the increase in nasal tip projection (see **Fig. 1**). Complete release of the lateral piriform is

necessary as well as circumferential release the caudal nasal bones via lateral, transverse, and green stick radix osteotomies. If the nasal bones are very short, then no bone cuts may be needed. In most cases, some small cartilage grafts or soft tissue (perichondrium) may be needed to set the supratip position and create a smooth dorsum. Costal perichondrium can also be used to attain small degrees of radix augmentation after the dorsum is elevated with an SDCG type A (**Fig. 9**; Video 3).

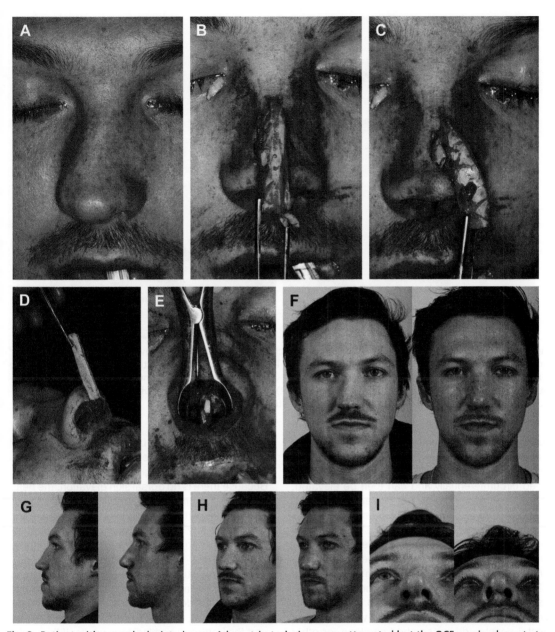

Fig. 8. Patient with severely deviated nose. A low strip technique was attempted but the QCF was inadequate to support the dorsum. The SDCG type B was used to salvage the operation. (*A*) Intraoperative frontal view showing severe deviation of the nose. (*B*) SDCG type B with attached native perichondrium. (*C*) SDCG with anterior curvature to enhance push up effect on the middle vault (*D*) Caudal septal replacement graft that was fixed to the nasal spine. (*E*) SDCG fixed to the caudal septal replacement graft. (*F*) Preoperative frontal view (left). Six-month postoperative frontal view (right). (*G*) Preoperative lateral view (left). Postoperative lateral view (right). (*H*) Preoperative oblique view (left). Postoperative oblique view (right). (*I*) Preoperative base view (left). Postoperative base view (right).

The width of the middle vault can be controlled by making the leading edge of the SDCG relatively narrow coming to a peak. In some cases, a trough can be made in the leading edge of the SDCG to accommodate remnant septum on the undersurface of the middle vault.

Patients who request larger degrees of dorsal augmentation and would like to have their radix elevated, can undergo placement of an SDCG type B with the cranial edge of the graft extending through the radix osteotomy site. In these cases, the nasal bones must be completely mobilized

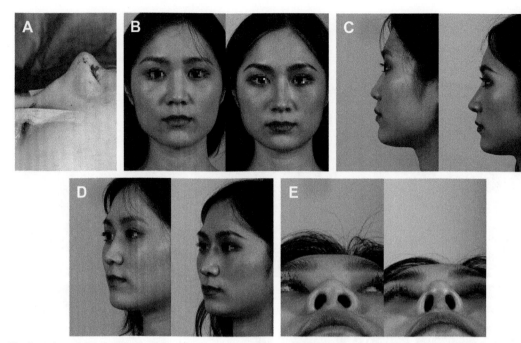

Fig. 9. Asian patient with a low dorsum and underprojected nasal tip. She desires elevation and narrowing of her dorsum and increased tip projection. (*A*) Intraoperative lateral view after tip projection was increased. Note the supratip depression. (*B*) Preoperative frontal view (left). One-year postoperative frontal view (right). (*C*) Preoperative lateral view (left). Postoperative lateral view (right). (*D*) Preoperative oblique view (left). Postoperative oblique view (right). (*E*) Preoperative base view (left). Postoperative base view (right).

through bilateral lateral osteotomies, bilateral transverse osteotomies, and a complete radix osteotomy. The bony and cartilaginous vaults are freed circumferentially and can then be elevated. Wide dissection of the periosteum around the piriform aperture and maxilla is necessary as well as complete release of the lateral keystone and division of the piriform ligament. Then the SDCG type B can be advanced through the radix osteotomy site to sit on top of the frontal bone. The SDCG is fixed to the nasal bones through a transosseous 4-0 PDS suture (Video 4). The superior end of the SDCG is camouflaged with a strip of costal perichondrium, crushed cartilage, or other soft tissue. The inferior end of the SDCG is fixed to a caudal septal extension graft that is fixed to the nasal spine. This creates a new L-shaped support structure to hold up the bony and cartilaginous vaults.

After completing the dorsal elevation, the airway should be assessed for any blockage due to the graft. If there is blockage, the inferior margins of the graft can be trimmed near the nasal valve. It is also helpful to place septal splints for a couple of weeks to help the septal flaps approximate.

One can also leave the dorsal nasal skin attached to the nasal dorsum and perform the entire push up from below the dorsum. The bone

cuts can be made from below and the small lateral wall stab incisions. The small camouflage grafts can be placed through the sidewall incisions. Because there is no dorsal skin elevation, the healing of the dorsum is maximized. Small depressions can be filled with autologous fat harvested at the time of surgery or finely diced cartilage particles injected with an 18-gauge needle along the nasal dorsum.

In order for the SDCG to support the bony and cartilaginous vaults, the costal cartilage should be dense and ideally partially calcified. If the costal cartilage is soft, it will not be strong enough to support the bony and cartilaginous vaults. If the costal cartilage is soft, then it is preferable to harvest a bone and cartilage costal cartilage segment (costochondral) with at least 50% bone and the rest cartilage. The bony end can be placed into the radix osteotomy site after contouring with a piezotome or bur. Then the cartilaginous end can be fixed to the caudal septal extension graft.

Patients with a low dorsum and low wide radix are ideal candidates for the SDCG type B (**Fig. 10**; Video 5). In these cases, the bony and cartilaginous vaults are freed up from the maxilla and frontal bone and septum. Then the SDCG type B is fashioned to extend through the radix osteotomy site and then integrate with the caudal

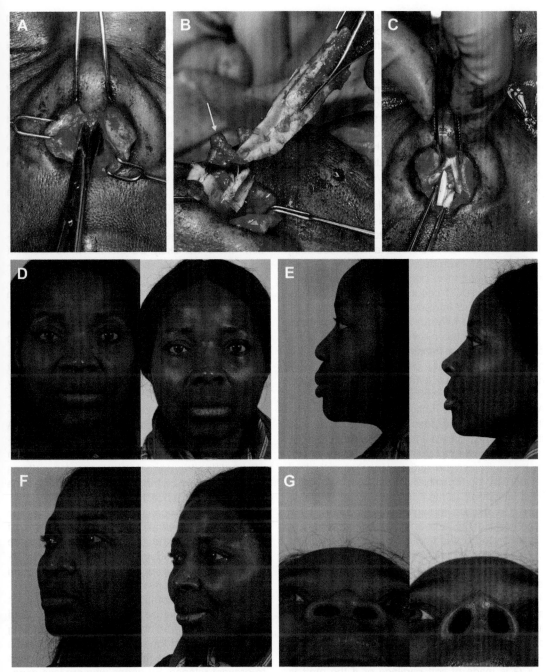

Fig. 10. Black patient with low dorsum and wide nose with wide nasal base and under projected tip. (*A*) Intraoperative view showing subdorsal cut to perform high strip and release of upper lateral cartilages from the septum. (*B*) SDCG type B carved with a platform to accommodate the nasal bones. The cranial extension extends through the radix osteotomy site to sit on the frontal bone. (*C*) Fixing the SDCG to the caudal septal extension graft. (*D*) Preoperative frontal view (left). One-year postoperative frontal view (right). (*E*) Preoperative lateral view (left). Postoperative lateral view (right). (*F*) Preoperative oblique view (left). Postoperative oblique view (right). (*G*) Preoperative base view (left). Postoperative base view (right).

septal extension graft. Ideally, there should be a high point along the graft (prominence) under the middle vault to insure adequate middle vault elevation.

DISCUSSION

The deficiencies of presently available techniques for dorsal augmentation are reflected in the numerous options for dorsal augmentation ranging from solid grafts to diced cartilage and fascia. Many of these methods have issues such as graft visibility, unnatural appearing dorsum, resorption, irregularities, and so forth. The major advantage of the SDCG is that most of the augmentation is accomplished by "pushing up" the bony and cartilaginous dorsum from below. Any fine tuning of the dorsal line is accomplished by placing smaller soft cartilage grafts or soft tissue grafts (costal perichondrium, fascia, scar tissue, crushed cartilage) on top of the dorsum. With smaller grafts or soft tissue over the dorsum, the possibility of deformity or visibility is relatively low.

Because the larger costal cartilage dorsal graft is below the dorsum, small defects or minor bending is less likely to affect dorsal contours. Additionally, the SDCG is carved in an axial (anterior–posterior) orientation to maximize strength of the segment and also to minimize bending.[5] While under the dorsum, the SDCG becomes encased under the bone and "locked" into position. Therefore, the likelihood of late deformity due to warping is decreased.

Radix augmentation is very difficult and tends to create an unnatural transition from radix to frontal process. Additionally, controlling proper radix height is also difficult. With the SDCG, it is easier to control the height of the radix. The SDCG type A provides very little radix augmentation, whereas the SDCG type B provides elevation dependent on the size of the cranial extension of the graft that extends through the radix osteotomy site. The height of the radix can be reduced postoperatively if needed by performing a "needle shave" under local anesthesia in the office setting. A 16-gauge needle is passed through the skin (under local anesthesia) of the radix and the cartilage segment sitting on top of the frontal bone can be shaved down to the appropriate height.

After augmenting the dorsum using an SDCG, it is apparent that bone forms in the gap between the nasal bones and the maxilla. This is due to the periosteum that is left along the gap between the nasal bones and maxilla. This adds significant stability to the pushed up dorsum. There can be some relapse and loss of dorsal height if the SDCG is made of soft cartilage or if the graft is not properly fixed to the caudal septal extension graft. The SDCG should be fixed to the nasal bones via a bone tunnel that can be drilled with 16-gauge needles. A 4-0 PDS suture passes through the holes and fixes to the SDCG. If proper fixation is not performed, then the SDCG can drift caudally and dislodge from the frontal bone. In some cases, the fixation can be performed to the stable frontal bone using a transcutaneous threaded Kirschner wire that can be removed in the office on the seventh postoperative day. The K-wire is advanced through a small dorsal stab incision and kept in the midline over the frontal process above the radix osteotomy site. This is a safe maneuver as long as the K-wire is kept in the midline.

Because the native nasal bones and upper lateral cartilages are left as the leading edge of the dorsum, the nasal bridge looks very natural. The width of the nasal dorsum can be controlled by the width of the leading edge of the SDCG. A wider leading edge will widen the dorsum and flare out the upper lateral cartilages and can provide a significant improvement in nasal breathing. The nasal bones have the capability to contour to the shape of the leading edge of the SDCG providing excellent narrowing in most cases.

With the increased popularity of dorsal preservation, there will likely be increased numbers of revision rhinoplasty cases requiring repair of deformities due to failed dorsal preservation operations. The SDCG can be used to correct deformities such as the "infantile radix" and saddle nose deformity. In the case of the infantile radix, the bone cuts can be revisited and the bony vault mobilized and then fixed into proper position using the SDCG type B. We have also used "tall spreader grafts" that extend to the radix area and extend above the low dorsum to correct the infantile radix with good success. The saddle deformity after dorsal preservation can also be corrected using the SDCG type A after releasing the lateral keystone and piriform ligament. Deviations noted after dorsal preservation will be difficult to correct using spreader grafts as the septum may be modified. Straightening of the nose can be accomplished using the SDCG.

Of key importance is the ability to salvage the failed dorsal preservation operation at the time of execution, using the SDCG. By stabilizing the collapsed support structures at the time of the surgery, complications such as the infantile radix and saddle nose deformity can be avoided.

The SDCG is a complex operation and requires a high level of expertise in dorsal preservation and costal cartilage grafting. An acute understanding of the anatomy of the osseous and cartilaginous vaults is required to accomplish adequate release to prevent relapse. Surgeons who are less experienced may choose to use "oblique spreader grafts" for saddle nose repair as a steppingstone to the SDCG. The oblique spreader grafts are sutured as an anterior extension off of the existing dorsal septum to "push up" the saddled middle vault.[4] These spreader grafts do not extend to the upper dorsal region, are limited to the area under the middle nasal vault and extend to the septal extension graft. This is a less complicated option for "pushing up" the saddled middle nasal vault.

FINAL COMMENTS

The SDCG has great utility in multiple forms of dorsal preservation. This unique graft has the capability to correct the saddle nose deformity, provide dorsal augmentation, and salvage failed dorsal preservation operations. This is a difficult operation and requires a high level of expertise in dorsal preservation and costal cartilage grafting.

CLINICS CARE POINTS

- SDCG can be used to correct the saddle nose deformity.
- SDCG can salvage a failed dorsal preservation operation.
- SDCG can elevate the low dorsum.
- SDCG type B can raise the radix and nasal dorsum.
- Strong rigid autologous costal cartilage is necessary for the SDCG.
- SDCG should be carved in an axial plane (anterior–posterior).
- SDCG type B extends through the radix osteotomy site.
- A full release of the piriform ligament and lateral keystone is necessary to avoid relapse.
- The SDCG must be fixed to the nasal bones to avoid caudal migration.
- A high point along the SDCG is needed under the upper lateral cartilages to adequately raise the middle vault.

SUPPLEMENTARY DATA

Supplementary data related to this article can be found online at https://doi.org/10.1016/j.fsc.2022.08.006.

REFERENCES

1. Daniel RK. The Preservation Rhinoplasty: A new rhinoplasty revolution. Aesth Surg J 2018;38:228–9.

2. Saban Y, Daniel RK, Polselli R, et al. dorsal preservation: the push down technique reassessed. Aesthet Surg J 2018;38(2):117–31.

3. Daniel RK, Palhazi P, Saban Y, et al. Preservation rhinoplasty. 3rd edition. Septum publishing; 2020.

4. Toriumi DM, Kovacevic M. Correction of the Saddle Nose Deformity Using the "Push Up" Technique. Facial Plast Surg 2022. https://doi.org/10.1055/a-1803-6341.

5. Toriumi DM. Subdorsal Cantilever Graft for Elevating the Dorsum in Ethnic Rhinoplasty. Facial Plast Surg Aesthet Med 2022;24(Number 3):143–59.

6. Ferraz MBJ, Zappelini CEM, Carvalho GM, et al. Cirurgia conservadora do dorso nasal—a filosofia do reposicionamento e ajuste do septo piramidal (SPAR). Rev Bras Cir Cabeca Pescoco 2013;42:124–30.

7. Ferriera MC. Spare roof technique. In Daniel RK, Palhazi P, Saban Y, et al, eds. Preservation rhinoplasty, 3rd ed., 2020, Septum publishing; Istanbul Turkey.

8. Toriumi DM. Lessons learned in thirty years of structure rhinoplasty. Chicago: DMT Solutions; 2019.

Brazilian Approach to Dorsum Preservation

Mario Bazanelli Junqueira Ferraz, MD[a], Wilson J. Dewes, MD[b], Luiz Carlos Ishida, MD, PhD[c], Guilherme Constante Preis Sella, MD, PhD[d],*

KEYWORDS

- Rhinoplasty • Dorsal preservation rhinoplasty • SPAR • Nasal deformity

KEY POINTS

- Neves Pinto and Ribeiro were the first Brazilians surgeons doing preservation rhinoplasty.
- Many have changed, and problems and counter indications were challenged, and solutions encountered.
- Brazilian preservation techniques are adopted and improved by many surgeons around the world.

INTRODUCTION

There is currently a rebirth of secular techniques, such as closed approach, dorsum preservation, conservative surgery of the dorsum, push down/let down, septal pyramidal adjustment and repositioning (SPAR), and many other names given during the last 120 years. It is time to look back, know, honor, give credits, and learn the innovations and mistakes from pioneers. As Churchill said: "The longer you look back, the farther you can look forward."

The history of dorsum preservation starts at the end of the nineteenth century, more specifically in 1899 when Joseph Lincoln Goodale published a paper entitled "A new method for operative correction of exaggerated Roman nose."[1] Dorsum preservation became more popular with Oliver Ames Lothrop and his paper in 1914: "An operation for correcting the aquiline nasal deformity. The use of a new instrument. Report of a case."[2] It reached its apex with the work of Maurice Cottle in the 1950s.[3,4]

Cottle noticed that the traditional removal of the nasal roof, described by Joseph,[5] could lead to aesthetic and functional sequelae; and he was the one who popularized the concept of preserving the nasal dorsum through many studies, articles,

and courses on his technique. Because of him and through many of his pupils, the concept or philosophy (as it is called in Brazil) spread around the world.

In Brazil these concepts arrived in the late 1960s and were stablished in the 1970s in Rio de Janeiro and São Paulo. Many names contributed to the growth of the philosophy in Brazil.

THE 1970S AND 1980S

The most important figure of this era was Roberto Neves Pinto, an otolaryngologist from Rio de Janeiro. He worked for most of his career on nasal physiology and function, has done courses, and was directly mentored by Maurice Cottle. He was the founder of the Brazilian Rhinology Society in 1974; during the time of his presidency, the aesthetic and functional surgery of the nose was promoted all over Brazil.

In 1971 he organized the first of many courses. It was titled "First Rhinoplasty Course with emphasis in Push Down." Invited attendees included Professor Dr Montserrat Villadiu from Barcelona and other push down surgeons. One of the students at that course was a young otolaryngologist called Wilson José Dewes.

[a] Department of Facial Plastic Surgery, Clinica Mario Ferraz, Campinas 87013-050, Brazil; [b] Department of Facial Plastic Surgery, FUNDEF and Clinica Wilson Dewes, Lajeado, Rio Grande do Sul, Brazil; [c] Plastic Surgery Division, University of São Paulo, São Paulo, Brazil; [d] Department of Facial Plastic Surgery, Clinica Sella, Maringa, Brazil
* Corresponding author. Av Cidade de Leiria, 600 - Centro – Maringa/PR Brazil 87013-280.
E-mail address: guilherme_sella@yahoo.com.br

Facial Plast Surg Clin N Am 31 (2023) 131–142
https://doi.org/10.1016/j.fsc.2022.08.010
1064-7406/23/© 2022 Elsevier Inc. All rights reserved.

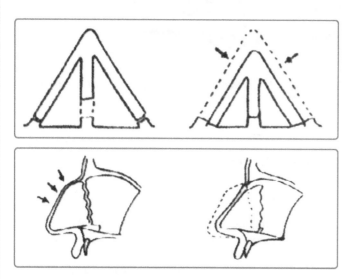

Fig. 1. Push down technique (*arrows*). (*Reproduced with minor modifications from* Neves Pinto RM. Rinossseptoplastia funcional. *Rev Bras Otorrinolaringol.* 1975;41(1):50 to 66.)

Neves Pinto published many studies, books, and articles on conservative surgery of the nose. In his article published in 1975 entitled "Functional Rhinoseptoplasty" he states: "The conservative surgery of the septum and pyramid, planned and executed by one surgeon, is a preservation surgery of the nasal tissues. All the structures are carefully mobilized, adjusted and economically reduced. Always accordingly with the golden rule: minimum of surgery and maximum result." He advocated maximal preservation of soft tissues, cartilage, and bone.[6]

In the same article he shows his approach at that time: using closed approach, through hemitransfixed septal incision, he corrects septal deviations, takes a low strip from the septum, and uses a push down osteotomy (**Fig. 1**).

Later in another publication[7] he describes the use of let down for the pyramid and two approaches for the septum, low with different designs to deal with the supratip area (**Figs. 2** and **3**), and describes his approach in deviated noses with asymmetrical osteotomies and let down (**Fig. 4**). There is no doubt that Neves Pinto was the number one surgeon in push down surgery during the 1970s and 1980s. Most of the otolaryngologists at that time learned the Cottle technique from him.

Liacyr Ribeiro, a plastic surgeon in Rio de Janeiro, presented his technique in 1978.[8] It was inspired in Cottle and Skoog. He makes a cut in the same level through upper lateral cartilages and septum, and the bone pyramid (**Fig. 5**). The upper part (where the hump is) is elevated and the lateral wall is diminished with rasps. As he gets the desired height he stops and lays the upper part (with the hump) on the lower part (the

basis). He also describes the same approach for deviated dorsum pushing the hump to the opposite side of the deviation (**Fig. 6**).

THE 1990S

During the 1990s the two main schools in preservation rhinoplasty emerged represented by Wilson José Dewes in Rio Grande do Sul and Jorge Ishida in São Paulo.

Jorge Ishida was born in 1939 to Japanese immigrants in Pompeia, São Paulo State. He graduated in medicine in 1963 and did his specialization in plastic surgery at São Paulo University, where he was head of the Nose Group of the University for more than 30 years. He taught his techniques to hundreds of residents in plastic surgery that passed through the Nose Group and Ishida Clinic.

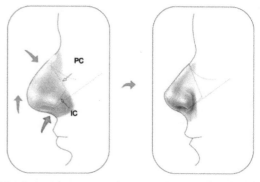

Fig. 2. Let down procedure. IC; PC. Reproduced with minor modifications from Neves Pinto RM. On the "let-down" procedure in septorhinoplasty. Rhinology. 1997;35(4):178 to 180. IC, inferior chondrotomy; PC, posterior chondrotomy.

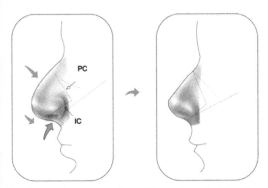

Fig. 3. Let down procedure. (*Reproduced with minor modifications from* Neves Pinto RM. On the "let-down" procedure in septorhinoplasty. Rhinology. 1997;35(4):178 to 180.)

He developed his version of the surgery inspired by traumatic cases. Observing some trauma patients who noted the appearance of their nose was improved after frontal trauma, he started to think of a procedure where he could keep the cartilaginous portion intact and work on the septum and the bone pyramid resecting it. It was the first

time in the literature an intermediate work in the septum was reported. Thus, the cartilaginous push down was born in the beginning of the 1990s and published in 1999.[9]

In this technique the cartilaginous framework is repositioned posteriorly and the osseous hump is removed. A transfixing incision is made, the perichondrium is elevated bilaterally, and the septum is exposed. A strip of cartilaginous septum is excised such that the width and the shape vary according to the amount of hump reduction desired. The cartilaginous septum is freed from the perpendicular plate of ethmoid as anteriorly as possible reaching the upper lateral cartilages. The dorsum is undermined through an intercartilaginous approach and the connection between cartilaginous and bone vaults is liberated and disconnected with blunt dissection. The cartilaginous hump is then pushed down without major resistance and stabilized into the new position with absorbable sutures in the cartilaginous septum. The osseous portion of the hump is removed at the same level of cartilaginous framework already positioned backward. A lateral osteotomy is performed to settle the nasal bones (**Figs. 7** and **8**).

Wilson José Dewes was born in 1939 to German and Italian immigrants in Arroio do Meio, State of Rio Grande do Sul. He graduated in 1963 from the Federal University of Santa Maria and specialized in anesthesiology. After a few years working as an anesthesiologist he became interested in otolaryngology. His most important mentor was Reinaldo Coser, professor in the university where he graduated. Coser performed Wilson Dewes' rhinoplasty, and because of this he became interested in this procedure and plastic surgery of the face.

In 1968 he started his practice in Lajeado, Rio Grande do Sul, and performed his first rhinoplasty. Three years later he went to Neves Pinto's course where he first heard about push down rhinoplasty. In 1982 he traveled as a visiting fellow to Barcelona to stay with Villadiu, the famous "Cottlelist." He also was influenced by many other push down professors, such as Ruben DeLuca from Buenos Aires, who he visited in 1990 and 1992.

In the late 1990s he performed push down on a regular basis after struggling for years with dorsum irregularities. The fact of living in a region where more than 90% of the population has German and Italian background contributed to the decision. "It was the only way I had in mind," says Wilson Dewes.

After few years experimenting with approaches, he developed his method to preserve the dorsum based on the low strip Cottle surgery. He called this technique reposicionamento e ajuste septo

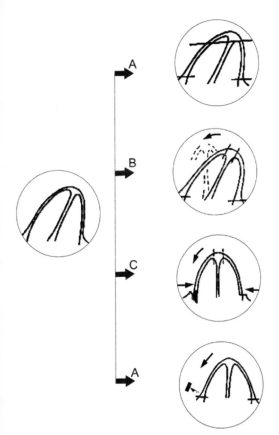

Fig. 4. Correcting the deviation of the nasal pyramid. (*Reproduced with minor modifications from* Neves Pinto RM. On the "let-down" procedure in septorhinoplasty. Rhinology. 1997;35(4):178 to 180.)

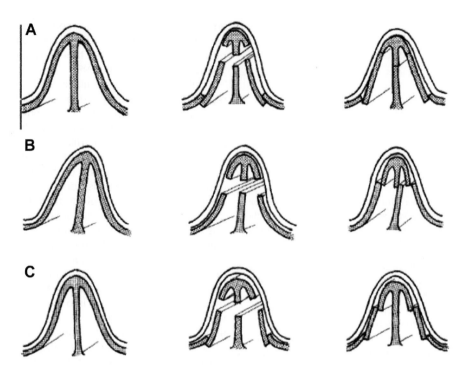

Fig. 5. Different levels of the fracture. (*A*) Cottle. (*B*) Incisions in different levels for deviations. (*C*) Incisions in different levels for reducing hump. (*Reproduced with minor modifications from* Ribeiro L. Rhinoplasty-A new approach in the repair of the hump. Aesthetic Plast Surg. 1978;2(1):409 to 418. https://doi.org/10.1007/BF01577979.)

piramidal, which was changed in 2005 by suggestion of a young surgeon who would become a follower and great adopter of the technique, Mario Ferraz from Campinas, São Paulo. The new name would be the English version, SPAR, because it sounds better and can explain in an anatomic way the SPAR technique.

In 1998 he organized his first course and demonstrated his technique in live surgeries. At that time 30% of his surgeries were already SPAR.

This technique consisted of:

1. Transfixing septal incision and subperichondrial undermining
2. Modification of the septum (types A, B, or C)
3. Modification of the pyramid; correct bony irregularities using rasps or motor devices and delicate reshaping of the cartilaginous pyramid without separating the upper lateral cartilages from the septum
4. Transverse osteotomies at the point of the new radix
5. Lateral osteotomies after subperiosteal detachment
6. Complete release of the pyramid from the face
7. Septopyramidal readjustment; movements include lateralization and anteroposterior repositioning (lowering or suspending the pyramid)

In April 2005 during Rhinology 2005/24th ISIAN in São Paulo Dr Yves Saban came to lecture and show his concepts in rhinoplasty. In the same room, speaking before Saban, Dewes presented his concepts, which matched 100% with Saban's concepts. Because of this unexpected meeting Dewes was introduced to Gola's technique, which consisted of a high horizontal cut 5 mm below the upper lateral cartilages and to push down the dorsum with an overlap between the septum above and below the cut is done.

It was perfect for patients who did not need to have the septum corrected. Less trauma could be avoided; the detachment of the septum from the corridor and perpendicular plate would not be necessary if the septum was already straight. The only problem with Gola's technique was because of the overlap a tilt of the dorsum could happen. Dewes decided to remove the cartilage above the horizontal cut in the septum and suture the two ends. Thus, another type of procedure was born. This "new" type of SPAR was named SPAR A (for alto, which means high in Portuguese; **Fig. 9**). The "old" version with the low cut in the septum was named SPAR B (for baixo, which means low in Portuguese; **Fig. 10**); and the push up became SPAR C (**Fig. 11**).

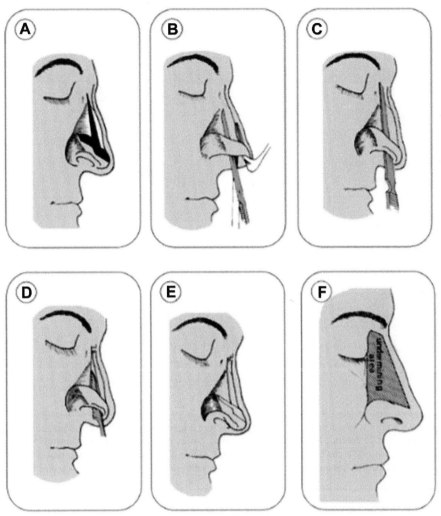

Fig. 6. (*A–F*) Surgical plan. (*Reproduced with minor modifications from* Ribeiro L. Rhinoplasty-A new approach in the repair of the hump. Aesthetic Plast Surg. 1978;2(1):409 to 418. https://doi.org/10.1007/BF01577979.)

SPAR C (push up) was always a challenge for Dewes. With a population of almost 100% Whites, Lajeado was not the best place to develop this technique. Push up was always a topic of discussion everywhere but there was no case of success until Dewes' first attempts.

In 2017 the first case of a SPAR C technique was done. All of the pyramid was released, and instead

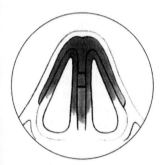
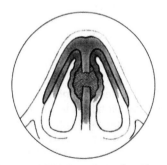
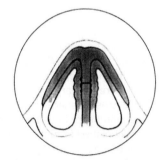

Fig. 7. Midportion of the cartilaginous hump and its lowering after the resection of a septal fragment. (Ishida, Jorge M.D.; Ishida, Luiz Carlos M.D.; Ishida, Luis Henrique M.D.; Vieira, José Cássio Rossi M.D.; Ferreira, Marcus Castro M.D.. Treatment of the Nasal Hump with Preservation of the Cartilaginous Framework. Plastic and Reconstructive Surgery: May 1999 - Volume 103 - Issue 6 - p 1729-1733.)

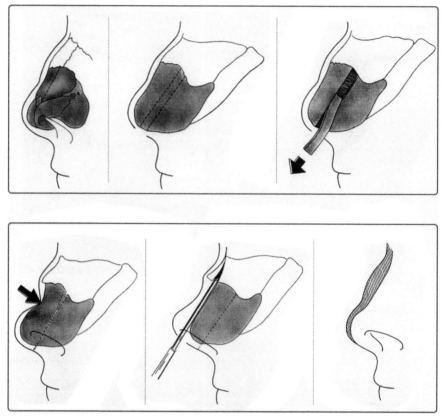

Fig. 8. Lateral view, excision of a strip of the cartilaginous septum, lowering of the cartilaginous hump, and resection of the osseous hump. (Ishida, Jorge M.D.; Ishida, Luiz Carlos M.D.; Ishida, Luis Henrique M.D.; Vieira, José Cássio Rossi M.D.; Ferreira, Marcus Castro M.D.. Treatment of the Nasal Hump with Preservation of the Cartilaginous Framework. Plastic and Reconstructive Surgery: May 1999 - Volume 103 - Issue 6 - p 1729-1733.)

of a wide undermining of the perichondrium only a small tunnel was done superiorly close to the roof. It was only possible to make the cuts in high septum and perpendicular plate; cartilage was harvested from the base of the septum (from an inferior tunnel not connected to the superior) and placed between the septum and the roof of the nose. The pyramid was then pushed up. To keep it in place a hard splint was kept in place bilaterally for 60 days (**Fig. 12**).

The second push up case was done in that same year in a patient that had history of trauma as a child. The SPAR B technique was performed, and during the septum deviation correction maneuver there was an increase of the height. Bone pyramid was pushed up supported with septal cartilage and kept in place supported with splints bilaterally placed from the floor of the nose to the roof for 60 days (**Fig. 13**).

The first decade of the 2000s was the period when these two techniques (SPAR and Ishida) were really established. They began to be taught frequently in courses, especially in Wilson Dewes'

courses, which were gaining more relevance among otolaryngologists, and in the State University of São Paulo by Ishida and sons among plastic surgeons.

Dr Perboyre Lacerda, professor in the Otolaryngology Department in State University of São Paulo, learned SPAR directly from Wilson Dewes and started to teach it in the residency program. Many other professors in the same university started to adopt the technique, especially Carlos Caropreso e José Roberto Parisi Jurado.

Alexandre Murta must be remembered as well. He was an otolaryngologist and plastic surgeon. He was a great disseminator of the SPAR technique learned from Wilson Dewes and started to teach it in the residency program where he was an instructor for otolaryngologists and plastic surgeons.

Suddenly many surgeons were familiar with the concept of preserving the dorsum and it spread everywhere in the country. Many adopted the technique. Surgeons who did not adopt it at least heard about it.

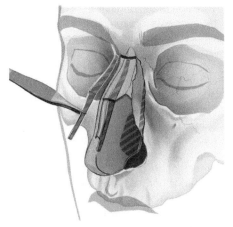
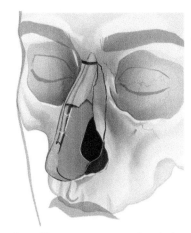

Fig. 9. SPAR A. *Hatched areas* in the septum and frontal process of maxilla area are removed and of potential use for grafting.

At the same time structured rhinoplasty gained popularity and started to be the state of the art because apparently it brought the solution for the hump removal sequelae. Critics of the techniques that preserve the dorsum claimed structured rhinoplasty was superior and there was no more space for the "archaic techniques." Rhinoplasty courses were the place for the dispute, often unfairly because critics of the preservation technique outnumbered the defenders. Just to give and idea it was comparable with the eternal question: closed versus open approach.

In 2009, invited by Mario Ferraz and Wilson Dewes, Yves Saban came for a hands-on course exclusively on preservation techniques. The two masters finally were together in the operating room. Dewes showed the two SPAR approaches and Saban showed his technique and osteotomies. The great discussion was about how to perform osteotomies. Saban informed that his dream was to make osteotomies more controlled and that a power machine that does not harm the soft tissues should be developed.

PRESENT GENERATION

The present resurgence of dorsum preservation must be devoted to the pupils of the two masters of the previous decades. Hundreds of surgeons became familiar with the techniques. Fewer performed them on a regular basis. Three must be mentioned for their contributions in the field,

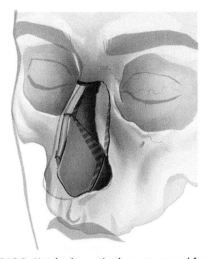
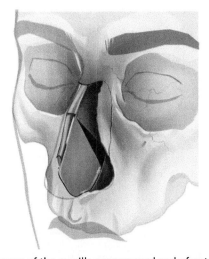

Fig. 10. SPAR B. *Hatched areas* in the septum and frontal process of the maxilla are removed and of potential use for grafting.

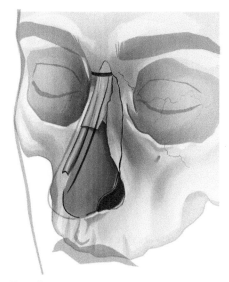

Fig. 11. SPAR C.

international relevance, and teaching over the years.

Luiz Carlos Ishida, Mario Ferraz, and José Carlos Neves

Luiz Carlos Ishida, born in 1968, son of Jorge Ishida, is a plastic surgeon in São Paulo. He graduated from Federal University of São Paulo in 1992 and is active as a professor for the residency program. With his brother, Luis Henrique Ishida, they continue to teach Ishida's technique and continue improving it. In 2020 he published a

variation of the original work. In this new approach he suggests preserving the bone cap to keep a smoother transition between the bone and cartilaginous middle third of the nose. In the same article he also showed a modification in the cut of the septum. He described a low cut (low strip) and a higher strip initiating close to w-point preserving completely the caudal septum (**Fig. 14**).[10]

In 2021, in a publication with Miguel Gonçalves Ferreira, they proposed another way to preserve bone cap. Instead of a triangular, a rectangular preservation of the bone cap is presented. The posterior border being the transverse osteotomy, lateral borders are osteotomies done at the level of brow-tip line. A wedge resection in a triangular shape is done laterally to the bone cap bilaterally. This is the amount of the descent of the bone pyramid at the level of the bone cap. The rest of the bone dorsum is sculptured, or lateral osteotomies are done to narrow the pyramid (**Fig. 15**).[11]

Mario Ferraz is an otolaryngologist and craniomaxillofacial surgeon in Campinas, State of São Paulo. Born in Campinas in 1977, he graduated from the State University of Campinas in 2001. In 2005 after finishing his residency program he spent 3 months in an internship program at Dewes Clinic where he learned the technique. By his suggestion the name was modified to SPAR. He then moved to Portland to be an international fellow in facial plastic surgery at Oregon Health and Science University under mentorship of Ted Cook and Tom Wang. There he met José Carlos Neves and invited him to come to Brazil and learn an innovative technique. In 2006 he visited Yves

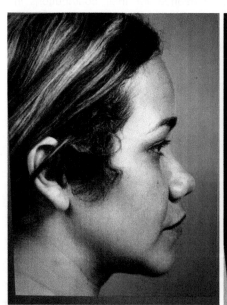
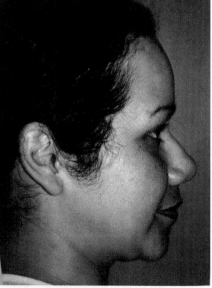

Fig. 12. Preoperative and postoperative of the first SPAR C technique performed by Dr Dewes (personal archive).

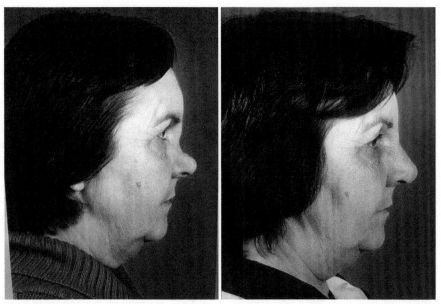

Fig. 13. Preoperative and postoperative of a SPAR C technique performed by Dr Dewes (personal archive).

Saban in Nice to learn with him and make the connection between the Saban and Dewes techniques. It culminated with the 2009 course in Lajeado and the 2012 course in Nice, both devoted to preservation techniques.

From 2007 to 2008 Ferraz worked with Dewes as his assistant and in 2009 he went back to Campinas to establish the facial plastic division in the otolaryngology discipline. From 2009 to 2015 the SPAR technique was the main technique used and taught by him to fellows, residents, and visitors.

In 2013 he standardized the variations of SPAR with precise indications. [12] It seems to be the first description in the literature setting the indications for high and low septal work, and the first to describe the technique for push up (SPAR C).

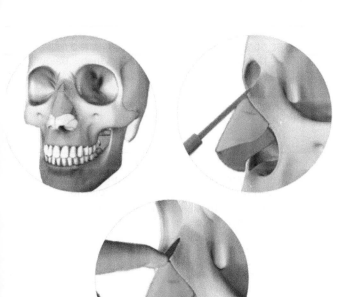

Fig. 14. Lowering the dorsum. (*From* Ishida LC, Ishida J, Ishida LH, Tartare A, Fernandes RK, Gemperli R. Nasal hump treatment with cartilaginous push-down and preservation of the bony cap. Aesthetic Surg J. 2020;40(11):1168-1178. doi:https://doi.org/10.1093/asj/sjaa061.)

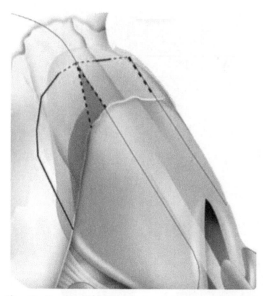

Fig. 15. Ferreira-Ishida technique: spare roof type B. (From Ferreira MG, Ishida LC, Ishida LH, Santos M. Ferreira-Ishida Technique: Spare Roof Technique B. Step-by-Step Guide to Preserving the Bony Cap while Dehumping. Plast Reconstr Surg. 2022;149(5):901E-904E. doi:https://doi.org/10.1097/PRS.0000000000009060.)

Type C is the subtype used to project the nasal pyramid. Preparation of the septum and pyramid is done as described for SPAR A but instead of lowering the pyramid it is projected using bone and cartilaginous grafts between the extremities of the septum and lateral bone walls with the goal to keep the pyramid suspended (**Table 1**).[12]

In 2021 he described the best indications for preservation techniques and the types of nose

that would not be the best indications for "pure" preservation techniques and thus should be avoided.[13] He described the preservation stigmas as low radix, wide middle third, residual or persistent hump, and saddling of the supratip area. He also suggested the methods to avoid complications and expand indications as fixation of the septum in a posterior position during SPAR B or low strips techniques, osteoplasty of the pyramid with piezoelectric instruments and drill and sculpture of the cartilaginous pyramid using electric cautery in cut mode, use of the ballerina maneuver in kyphotic dorsums, and onlay grafts in the radix or supratip areas.[13] He also revisited SPAR technique in another article in 2021 with Dewes and Neves.[14]

José Carlos Neves was born in Coimbra, Portugal in 1974 and graduated from Coimbra University in 1998. He learned the SPAR technique during his internship at the Dewes Clinic in 2007. He took all the concepts to Europe and disseminated the ideas based on the SPAR philosophy. In 2019 described the technique inspired in SPAR A with modification in the height and shape of the cut in the septum.[15] He also explained how the shape of the dorsum could be modified using vertical cuts in the higher segment. It was important to expand the indications for SPAR A and other high strip techniques (**Fig. 16**).[15]

The same year he published an evolution of the previous technique.[16] The goal was to make the segments more stable by leaving the caudal border of the septum intact and use it as an additional fixation point. In this technique a rectangular piece of cartilage is designed below the

Table 1
SPAR classification and characteristics of the subtypes

	A	B	C
Technical characteristics	High septal strip	Disinsertion from the premaxilla corridor and PPE	Hight septal approach and use of grafts to keep projection
Indications	Narrow nose with straight septum, without kyphotic appearance of dorsal irregularities	Lowering of the nasal pyramid + correction of deviated nasal septum + laterorhinia + kyphotic nose	Project the nasal pyramid
Contraindications or need for mixed techniques	Severe irregularities and kyphotic dorsum	Wide nasal dorsum; severe irregularities and complex high dorsum	Nasal pyramids that need big projection

Abbreviation: PPE, perpendicular ethmoidal plate.

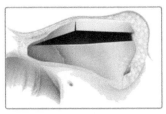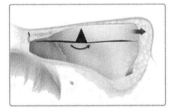

Fig. 16. The Vitruvian man. (© Fernando Vilhena de Mendonca. From Neves JC, Arancibia Tagle D, Dewes W, Larrabee W. The split preservation rhinoplasty: "the Vitruvian Man split maneuver." Eur J Plast Surg. 2020. doi:https://doi.org/10.1007/s00238-019-01600-3.)

cartilaginous hump in between the most prominent point of the hump and caudal border of the upper lateral cartilages (W point). Two vertical lines measuring 5 to 8 mm are designed perpendicular to the dorsum at the level of the upper lateral cartilages caudal border (caudal border of the rectangle). The second line is at the level of the most

prominent point of the hump (cephalic border). A line is made uniting the two previous ones; the Tetris block is done. Resection of cartilage around the block is made to open space for the descent of the block and consequently the dorsum. The great advantage of the technique is the possibility to stabilize the block in two vectors, vertical and

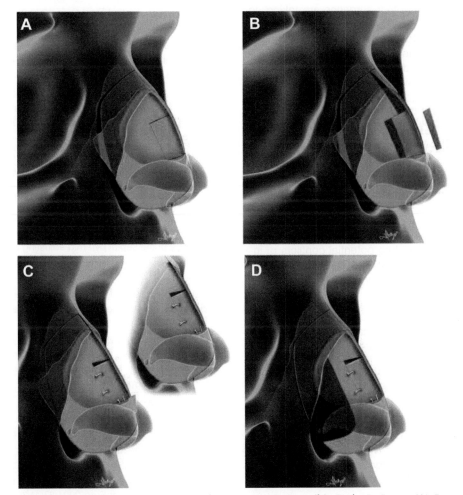

Fig. 17. (*A–D*) Split Tetris concept. (*Reproduced from* Neves JC, Arancibia-Tagle D, Dewes W, Ferraz M. The Segmental Preservation Rhinoplasty: The Split Tetris Concept. Facial Plast Surg. 2021;37(1):36–44. https://doi.org/10.1055/s-0040-1714672.)

horizontal, and avoid recurrence and tilting of the pyramid (**Fig. 17**).[16]

SUMMARY

Brazil has always been a fertile place for plastic surgery techniques, especially cosmetic, and it was not different in rhinoplasty. As we review the history of the techniques of preservation, we realize much was developed in the country. Even with the loss of popularity of the preservation technique it was never abandoned and has always been present and taught. SPAR and Ishida's techniques have evolved during the last decade especially in recent years with the renaissance of preservation. Problems and contraindications were challenged, and solutions encountered. As a result, indication was expanded to almost every kind of nose. Surface work was executed with power tools, such as the piezoelectric device and drill, and came to complement and to refine. In recent years many other surgeons are taking up nasal dorsum preservation with a variety of new techniques; unfortunately, we cannot name them all here. Today the Brazilian preservation techniques are adopted and improved by many surgeons around the world.

CLINICS CARE POINTS

- Review of the history of rhinoplasty in Brazil

DECLARATION OF CONFLICTING INTERESTS

The authors declared no potential conflicts of interest with respect to the research, authorship, and/or publication of this article.

FUNDING

The authors received no financial support for the research, authorship, and/or publication of this article.

DISCLOSURE

The authors have nothing to disclose.

ACKNOWLEDGMENTS

The authors acknowledge authors Neves Pinto, Ribeiro, and Ishida for the use of their figures under the public domain.

REFERENCES

1. Goodale J. A new method for the operative correction of the exaggerated roman nose. Bost Med Surg J 1899;140:112.

2. Lothrop OA. An operation for correcting the aquiline nasal deformity; the use of a new instrument; report of a case. Bost Med Surg J 1914;170(22):835–7.

3. Cottle MH. Nasal roof repair and hump removal. AMA Arch Otolaryngol 1954;60(4):408–14.

4. Cottle MH. 1900 to 1910; a brief survey and bibliography. AMA Arch Otolaryngol 1958;67(3):327–33.

5. Joseph J. Nasenplastik und sonstige Gesichtsplastik. Leipzig: Curt Kabitzsch; 1931.

6. Neves Pinto RM. Rinosseptoplastia funcional. Rev Bras Otorrinolaringol 1975;41(1):50–66.

7. Neves Pinto RM. On the "let-down" procedure in septorhinoplasty. Rhinology 1997;35(4):178–80.

8. Ribeiro L. Rhinoplasty: a new approach in the repair of the hump. Aesthet Plast Surg 1978;2(1):409–18.

9. Ishida J, Ishida LC, Ishida LH, et al. Treatment of nasal hump with preservation of the cartilaginous framework. Plast Reconstr Surg 1999;103(6):1729–33.

10. Ishida LC, Ishida J, Ishida LH, et al. Nasal hump treatment with cartilaginous push-down and preservation of the bony cap. Aesthet Surg J 2020;40(11):1168–78.

11. Ferreira MG, Ishida LC, Ishida LH, et al. Ferreira-ishida technique: spare roof technique B. Step-by-step guide to preserving the bony cap while dehumping. Plast Reconstr Surg 2022;149(5):901E–4E.

12. Ferraz MBJ, Zappelini CEM, Carvalho GM De, et al. Conservative surgery of the nasal dorsum: the philosophy of the septal pyramid adjusting and repositioning (S.P.A.R.). Rev Bras Cir Cabeça Pescoço 2013;42(3):124–30.

13. Ferraz MBJ, Sella GCP. Indications for preservation rhinoplasty: avoiding complications. Facial Plast Surg 2021;37(1):45–52.

14. Dewes W, Zappelini CEM, Ferraz MBJ, et al. Conservative surgery of the nasal dorsum: septal pyramidal adjustment and repositioning. Facial Plast Surg 2021;37(1):22–8.

15. Neves JC, Arancibia Tagle D, Dewes W, et al. The split preservation rhinoplasty: "the Vitruvian Man split maneuver. Eur J Plast Surg 2020. https://doi.org/10.1007/s00238-019-01600-3.

16. Neves JC, Arancibia-Tagle D, Dewes W, et al. The segmental preservation rhinoplasty: the split Tetris concept. Facial Plast Surg 2021;37(1):36–44.

Ultrasonic Rhinoplasty and Septoplasty for Dorsum Preservation and for Dorsum Structural Reconstruction

Olivier Gerbault, MD

KEYWORDS

- Ultrasonic rhinoplasty • Ultrasonic septoplasty • Dorsum preservation
- Dorsum structural reshaping • Piezoelectric instruments • Piezotome • Nose ostectomies
- Rhinosculpture • Preservation rhinoplasty • Push Down • Let Down

KEY POINTS

- Ultrasonic rhinoplasty and septoplasty is the use of piezoelectric instruments (PEI) to perform the bone work during rhinoplasty and septoplasty. It is used in Preservation Rhinoplasty and in Structural Rhinoplasty.
- PEI are gentle instruments selective on bones and hard cartilages, that never create unwanted fracture or comminution, and preserve bone stability, unlike blunt force instruments (osteotomes, rasps)
- PEI allow the safe use of a full open or closed approach allowing the visualization of the whole bony vault to perform osteotomies, ostectomies and rhinosculpture.
- Ultrasonic rhinoplasty and septoplasty ease dorsum preservation by controlling the osteotomies and ostectomies for foundation techniques, osteotomies and rhinosculpture for surface techniques, and the bony septal trimming for high, intermediate and low strips.
- Ultrasonic rhinoplasty and septoplasty allow to control and smoothen the osseocartilaginous dorsum when structural reshaping of the dorsum is performed after hump removal, avoiding in most cases the use of concealment graft in the keystone areas.

INTRODUCTION

Preservation rhinoplasty has gained a significant popularity in recent years. Preservation of the dorsum is one of the key sequences of many preservation rhinoplasties.[1] It most often consists in lowering the cartilaginous or osseocartilaginous roof while preserving its central structure. To achieve such lowering, it is necessary to weaken this septotriangular pyramid (STP) by acting on the underlying structures that support it:

- The nasal septum
- The connections between the upper lateral cartilages (ULC) and the nasal bones, often improperly called ligaments, and also the pyriform attachments

- The nasal bones (nasal proper bone and ascending branch of the maxilla)

The precise control of this lowering results from the way in which the support structures of the STP are weakened and from the stabilization of the STP in its new position.

In some cases, however, the profile line should not be changed. This usually involves decreasing the width of the bone pyramid and/or STP. Because no lowering is planned, the support structures must be preserved.

Finally, the dorsum is raised when the profile line must be moved forward. The support structures of the STP must be interrupted to increase its projection thanks to elevation spreader grafts positioned higher than usual on the septum. The whole

Plastic Surgery, PEMV, 3 Cours Marigny, Vincennes 94300, France
E-mail address: dr.gerbault@gmail.com

Facial Plast Surg Clin N Am 31 (2023) 143–154
https://doi.org/10.1016/j.fsc.2022.09.002
1064-7406/23/© 2022 Elsevier Inc. All rights reserved.

dorsum can be raised, or only the lower part of it to lift the supratip area of the dorsum, depending on the length and the placement of the spreader grafts.

Bone preservation, in its integrity and in its attachments with the ULC, is an important element of stability in the immediate and long term. Bone stability, however, prevents the development of bone lowering for impaction techniques. This bone stability is directly dependent on the width and length of the cut bone flap, the persistence of connections with adjacent bones and cartilages, the preservation of the support structures of these bones (underlying periosteum and mucosa), and finally the reconstitution of bone stabilization when necessary.

Regarding the bone and cartilaginous structures of the nose, there are three actors to consider:

1. Bones and cartilage
2. The instruments used
3. The surgeon

BONES AND CARTILAGE

It is easy to assess the characteristics of cartilage by touch or by using instruments. The fineness, flexibility, and elasticity of cartilage plays an important role in the cartilage reshaping techniques used (eg, trimming, sutures, sliding flaps, support grafts), and the shape and position of these cartilages.

However, it is impossible to evaluate the same characteristics of nasal bones without piezoelectric instruments (PEI). A piezoelectric saw and a piezo rasp give an immediate feedback on the hardness of the bone and its thickness. From the first osteotomy performed, one can evaluate the flexibility and elasticity of the bones. These parameters have important consequences on the type of osteotomies to be performed, if those osteotomies are complete or partial, the location of osteotomies, and the association with a more or less extensive rhinosculpture.[2,3]

Schematically, for hard bones, osteotomies need to be more extensive and generally complete so that the bones can move properly. The saw should be oriented in a more sagittal way so that the obliquity of the cutting line allows the bones to move more easily. It is eventually necessary to be a little higher by 1 mm laterally and lower cephalically to allow the bones to move more easily. Conversely, for thin bones, partial osteotomies are usually sufficient except in some cases of very wide bone pyramid, because these thinner bones move much more easily. A more horizontal cut may be desirable to preserve some bone

stability. In case of very flexible and elastic bones, it may be necessary to use a bone wedge in the fracture line of the lateral osteotomies to prevent the bones from spreading or coming out in case of impaction. Brittle bones require the realization of complete osteotomies to avoid unwanted fractures.

In case of foundation techniques, lateral, transverse and medial osteotomies are mandatory, with additional ostectomy of the webster triangle and eventually part of the sidewalls for Let Down. The impaction is easy in case of thin bones. Conversely in case of thick bones, the ostoeotomy location should be 1 mm more medial for the lateral osteotomies and 1 mm more caudal for the transverse and root osteotomies.

THE INSTRUMENTS USED

The specificities of PEI are as follows:[4]

- To perfectly control the position and path of the fracture lines without causing any unwanted or radiated fractures. These osteotomies are made under complete visual control as soon as an extended open or closed approach is performed.
- To preserve the supporting force of the underlying structures (ULC, periosteum, mucosa, osseocartilaginous attachments or ligaments) because of their selectivity.
- To allow the realization of rhinosculpture, that is a progressive abrasion of the bony cap. This rhinosculpture changes bone biomechanics by making the bone flexible at first while maintaining its integrity. If continued, all the bony cap is removed but ULC are preserved, and the osseocartilaginous attachments. This rhinosculpture is essential in the areas of the dorsal and lateral keystone for the structural reconstruction of the dorsum, but also for cartilaginous impaction techniques and as a complementary gesture to be performed on a persistent bone hump during push down/ let down techniques.
- To allow to mobilize and orient the nasal bones in a precise way according to the position and the path of the osteotomy, and eventually the use of bone sutures (simple to perform in a full open approach after using an ultrasonic drill to drill holes from each part of the fracture line), and the use of grafts in the osteotomy line.

These instruments must be used gently by constantly cooling the working area of the insert thanks to the integrated irrigation, which must be set to at least 60 mL/minute. Therefore, the use of a suction retractor is highly recommended so as not to be bothered by water. There are 2 types of suction retractors: one for open ultrasonic rhinoplasty and the other for closed ultrasonic rhinoplasty, or when only a tunnel is developped on the bony sidewalls without central undermining of the skin. Suction speculum of dierent leght exist also for ultrasonic septoplasty. It is undesirable to press the bones with these instruments. Each insert requires a certain gesture to optimize its use.

It is also important to note that not all piezoelectric motors (units) are similar in their characteristics and in their power or in the use attributed to them. For example, many piezo units are designed solely for dental use and do not have approval for use in the operating room. Inserts designed for maxillofacial surgery are thicker and wider because they are intended to cut a much denser and thicker maxillary bone than the nasal bones. The defect at the cutting line is then greater, with a more prolonged bone healing and especially an increased risk of bone instability, but also a risk of bone defect perception in the areas where the overlying skin is thin. These inserts are resterilizable five times. Then they can wear out and be less effective, in the same way that an osteotome wears out. An osteotome can be sharpened, which is not the case for PEI.

The inserts for rhinoplasty are as follows: (1) short inserts more specifically for open ultrasonic rhinoplasty (**Figs. 1–6**), (2) long inserts more specifically for closed ultrasonic rhinoplasty and ultrasonic septoplasty **Figs. 7–11**.

THE SURGEON

PEI allows inexperienced surgeons to achieve nearly the same degree of precision in bone surgery and septum surgery as experts. It is indisputable that it takes some experience to obtain reliable and reproducible results in nose bone surgery. However even the most experimented surgeons can't be aware of the bone biocharacteristics before the surgery. Therefore, they can't adapt the type of osteotomies, ostectomies and the use of rhinosculpture to those characteristics. Finally, even experts can hardly control accurately the bone movements, final position and orientation if a full open or closed approach is not used.

THE DIFFERENT TECHNIQUES OF PRESERVATION OF THE DORSUM WITH PIEZOELECTRIC INSTRUMENTS

For all these techniques, the extensive subperiosteal dissection of the bone pyramid in its entirety allows a perfect visualization of the anatomic variations of the bones, but also of the osteotomies. It also makes it possible to combine on all parts of the pyramid osteotomies, ostectomies, and rhinosculpture to precisely reshape the bone pyramid. This extensive degloving of the bony vault, called full open approach or full closed approach (4) allows also to controle precisely bone mobilization and orientation, but also stabilization with sutures and grafts placed in the osteotomy site. The only drawback of the full open or closed approaches is an increased swelling in the following post-operative weeks that can be decreased by appropriate per and post op medications and taping, but also by an extended bone abrasion with the rasps to create a good skin adhesion.

Osteotomies are done by some surgeons through small tunnels endonasally or even percutaneous, but with a significant risk of bone and skin burn. An abundant cooling of the skin and of the bones with cold saline must then be

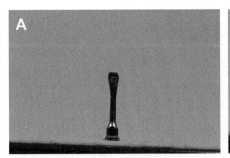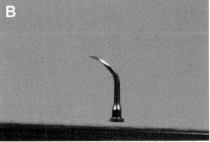

Fig. 1. (*A, B*) Scraper (RHS1). This instrument is the most aggressive of all. It is intended to make ostectomies. Its use is primarily reserved for areas where the bones are very thick and dense, such as the radix and the central part of the bony hump, the side walls. Its use in areas where the bones are not very thick should be careful to avoid creating bone defects. The incorrectly used scraper can damage the ULC: this is an additional reason to switch to rasping when most of the bone has already been removed in the treatment of a bone hump. The scraper is especially useful in case of strong, high, wide radix. It is also useful in the initial treatment of a pronounced hump, especially when the bones are thick. It is also used when a global bony vault rhinosculpture is performed.

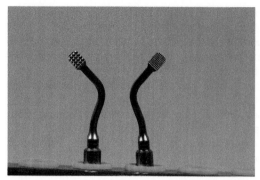

Fig. 2. Strong rasp (RHS2H) and fine rasp (RHS2F). Rasps are very soft instruments that allow one to make rhinosculpture. It abrases gradually the bony cap, which gradually modifies the biomechanical characteristics of the bones. Bones gradually become moldable and shapeable with rhinosculpture. In addition, sutures are passed through the refined bones in some cases, depending on the characteristics of the bones. Finally, these rasps do not damage the ULC. Rasps are essential in most cases of hump treatment, whether it is preservation or structural remodeling of the hump. They enable removal of the bony film from the lateral and dorsal keystone regions in a precise and atraumatic way for the underlying cartilages, thus allowing the anatomic reconstruction of the middle third or the lowering of the STP.

performed. Therefore external piezo ostoeotomies should be done very cautiously.

Bone Impactions (Push Down)

Piezoelectric saws allow a perfectly controlled shift downward of the bony pyramid under direct vision, whether it is an open or closed approach. The saws used are usually the thickest (RHS3 L and R), because they cause a slightly more significant defect at the fracture line facilitating bone sliding downward. The orientation of the saws for lateral osteotomies is more sagittal to promote bone sliding at this level.

Osteotomies are located 1 to 2 mm inside the nasofacial groove for lateral osteotomies, and 1 to 2 mm under the cephalic edge of the bones of the nose for transverse and root osteotomies, depending of the bone thickness as mentioned previously. These are areas where the bones are usually thick and move less easily than if these same osteotomies are performed closer to the piriform orifice (ie, more medially and lower), but this localization gives a little more stability and control over the movement of the bones, and also avoids deformations stair step deformity at the osteotomies.

The lateral osteotomy is started at the cephalic part of the Webster triangle, that is to say a little higher than for the usual lateral osteotomies, so as to avoid a blocking point at this level. For the same reason, the junction between the lateral osteotomy and the transverse osteotomy is rounded and not at a right angle.

To keep a more stable central hinge at the root, it is better to use thinner saws on the most medial part of the transverse osteotomies and for radix osteotomy. The high osteotomy of the perpendicular plate of the ethmoid (PPE) performed with the long saw joins the radix osteotomy started on either side of it, to bevel the radix osteotomy and avoid a collapse of the radix or a step deformity. In other wirds, the radix ostoeotmy is begun on both sides by sawing through the superficial aspect of the bone, and ended from inside with the long piezo saw in continuation with the PPE osteotomy. This PPE osteotomy is always necessary because the radix osteotomy is always located high (very cephalic) on the bone pyramid.

The sequence of osteotomies is performed before septum resections because there is no radiated fracture in ultrasonic rhinoplasty. This

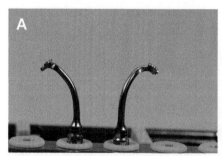
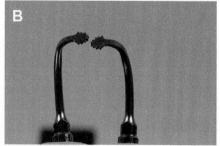

Fig. 3. (*A, B*) Saws for right lateral osteotomies (RHS3L) and left (RHS3R). The saws for lateral osteotomies have a design that allows to simply start the osteotomy very low in the area of the Webster triangle and follow the nasofacial groove to its upper edge. They are a little thicker than the other saws because the ascending branch of the maxilla is usually much thicker. They are preferred for lateral and transverse osteotomies for bone impaction techniques, because they create a greater defect on the fracture lines allowing a more marked slippage of the nasal bones.

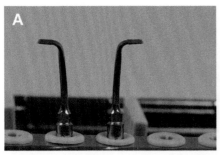
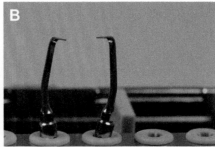

Fig. 4. (*A, B*) Saws for transverse osteotomies right (RHS4L) and left (RHS4R). Saws for transverse osteotomies are thinner, because they are intended to cut thinner bones (the nasal proper bones, the bony septum). They are also used in foundation impaction techniques for root osteotomies, which are complete or incomplete depending on whether one wishes to keep a median bone hinge or not.

allows one to assess, thanks to the piezo, the hardness or flexibility of the bones, and their ability to move more or less easily. Thus the resections of the septum have to be more cautious in case of very mobile bones, and conversely more marked in case of very stable thick bones.

In some cases of a wide bone pyramid, a paramedian or oblique median osteotomy may be added to reduce this bony width. This osteotomy is safely possible thanks to the strong support of the nasal bones provided by the periosteum and the mucosa, which are preserved under the nasal bones.

Finally, rhinosculpture is frequently combined with the osteotomies previously described to correct persistent bone convexities, but also to weaken the osteocartilaginous junction of the dorsal keystone to help flatten the top of the hump. This rhinosculpture with the rasps can be carried out at the beginning, but also after osteotomies, even on fully mobile bones.

In addition, these osteotomies performed before septum surgery make it possible to lift the roof of the STP to visually control perfectly the septum osteotomies once the first septal cut is made.

This septum surgery is thus made more precise and easier thanks to the visualization of the entire septum. The absence of a radiated fracture at the skull base allows the realization of safe osteotomies and ostectomies at the cephalic part of the PPE, which are often necessary to correct high septal deviations. Those osteotomies and ostectomies prevent an overlap of the deviated PPE from creating an axis deviation of the bone pyramid.

Another important advantage of long PEI is to allow the harvesting of significant intact pieces of osteocartilaginous septum for the purpose of supporting grafts even when a high strip is performed. Indeed in these cases, the Killian septal L ensuring the maintenance of the septum is shifted downward. The extended septal harvesting may weaken the stability of this septal L. This is even more true when a septum flap connected to the septotriangular roof is made to lower the latter in the Tetris technique[5] and in the Z flap.[6]

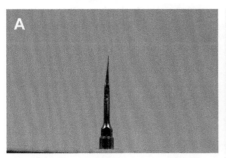
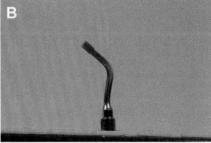

Fig. 5. The straight saw for median and paramedian osteotomies (RHS5). These saws are as thin as possible to perform osteotomies especially in places where the overlying skin is thin, so that the osteotomy is not noticeable. This is the case for median or paramedian osteotomies. But these saws are used for very fine bone cuts, such as when the bone on the impacted hump fragment is kept and/or when an osteotomy is performed in the area of the lateral keystone as in the Ishida technique. It is also used to make controlled ostectomies in let down techniques or when crisscross osteotomies are done to flatten convex bones. It is also useful for osteotomies or ostectomies of the nasal septum in the treatment of septal deviations, vomerian spurs.

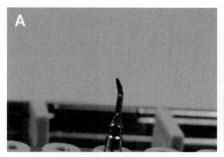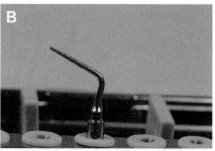

Fig. 6. (*A, B*) The drill to pierce the bones (RHS6). The drill is used to make holes in the bones, to suture bones to each other, or to puncture bones that are used to support cartilage. These sutures allow one to control the position of the nasal bones, but also to stabilize unstable bones, or to secure the nasal septum to the nasal spine or the nasal bones.

Finally, the extended open or closed approach allows the simple use of wedge sustain grafts in the caudal part of the lateral osteotomies, to stabilize the bones and secure the new position of the nasal bones, therefore avoiding any lateral movement of the bony vault. This approach allows also the simple use of various sutures between the ULC and the remaining septal strut to stabilize the STP in its new position.

Bone Lowering (Let Down)

The principles are the same as for bone impactions, except that an ostectomy is performed on the most caudal portion of the ascending branch of the maxilla to remove part of the Webster triangle to avoid any blocking point at this level. This ostectomy is performed either with a small straight saw or with the scraper. Unlike gouge ostectomies, ostectomies with PEI are easily done regardless of the thickness and density of the bones.

Some surgeons do more extensive ostectomies of the sidewalls to ease the lowering of the bony vault. However this maneuver may create a long term weakness of the bony vault.

Otherwise, the sequence is the same as for push down except bone stabilization, which cannot be performed.

Cartilage Impactions

PEI plays an important role here to perfectly smooth the nasal bones on the area of the lateral keystone (where a bony cartilaginous disjunction is performed), but also to cut precisely the bone fragment left possibly intact on the area of the dorsal keystone (Ishida technique).[4] Small ostectomies are also performed with a thin saw on the area of the lateral keystone in the Ferreira-Ishida technique.[7,8]

The perfect smoothing of the nasal bones is a crucial point in these surface techniques, where

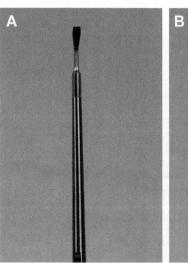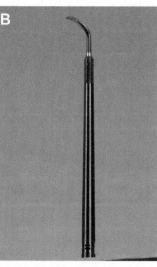

Fig. 7. (*A, B*) The long scraper. Like the short scraper, it allows ostectomies to be performed through a closed access, especially on the upper part of the nose.

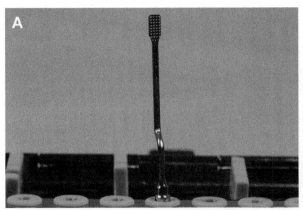
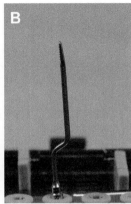

Fig. 8. (*A, B*) The long rasp. It allows the bone to be rasped down by closed approach on all parts of the bone pyramid. It is also used to correct a small residual bone hump during a touch up: a simple tunnel made internally enables one to reach the area to be treated and to rasp the residual bony hump without damaging the adjacent tissues.

unlike foundation techniques, an osseocartilaginous disjunction is performed on an area where the skin is usually thin. Piezo rasps are an indispensable tool to ensure a smooth transition and avoid bone roughness. Thanks to those rasps, concealment grafts are rarely necessary in the keystone area.

The Reductions in Width of the Osseocartilaginous Pyramid Without Modification of Height

In some cases, a reduction in the overall width of the nose is necessary without having to change the profile line by more than 1 mm. It is then possible to perform complete osteotomies with piezo: low lateral osteotomies, paramedian osteotomies, and transverse osteotomies. The peculiarity is that the paramedian osteotomy is performed without opening the middle third with a small straight saw (RHS5).

If the STP is still a little wide, several possibilities are available:

- Resect the cartilaginous corners (or shoulders) at the junction with the bone when they are protruding, which causes a prominent appearance on the oblique views. This maneuver can, however, generate residual defects if these cartilaginous corners are pronounced or if the overlying skin is thin. In these cases it is preferable to open the middle third to fold in the ULC to reshape the cartilaginous prominence.

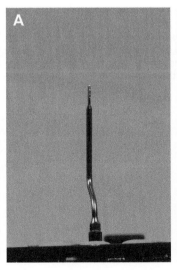
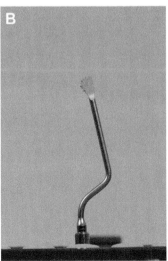

Fig. 9. (*A, B*) The straight long saw. It is intended to perform lateral and paramedian osteotomies by closed approach. Its length makes it possible to reach the most cephalic part of those osteotomies. It also plays an important role for osteotomies of the bony septum, whether in septoplasty, septum harvesting, or septum resections as part of dorsum preservation. For this last point, the long saw precisely cuts and trims the perpendicular plate of the ethmoid (PPE), but can also cut from below the nasal bones at the radix, allowing a beveled cut of the radix intended to allow a sliding of the bone downward rather than a sinking of the root in bone impaction techniques.

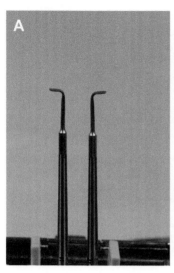
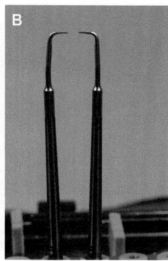

Fig. 10. (*A, B*) The right and left curved long saw. These two saws make it possible to perform transverse osteotomies by closed route, and osteotomies of the root by closed route in bone impaction techniques. They are also used for posterior osteotomies of the septum as part of septoplasty, septal harvesting, and septum cuts for dorsum preservation, especially for low strips.

- Partially incise the ULC over their entire height at the level of the desired dorsal aesthetic line, which attenuates the cartilage spring and reduces the width of the middle third.
- Perform U-shaped sutures with prolene at the top of the cartilaginous vault when the triangular cartilages are not weak (which would create cartilaginous deformations) to reduce the width of the middle third.

The Elevations of the Osteocartilaginous Pyramid (Push Up)

The osseocartilaginous pyramid is generally raised by performing the same osteotomies as in a push down, but by raising it thanks to spreader grafts positioned higher than normal, which allows this elevation.[9] PEI makes it easier to perform very high transverse and root osteotomies, to avoid the occurrence of a stair step when the bony pyramid is ascended.

The long piezo saw also makes it possible to carry out a precise incision of the PPE at its highest part, without the risk of radiated fracture, to allow the ascent of the pyramid.

Segmental elevation of the STP can be made to prevent or treat a supra tip saddling, i.e. when the supratip is too low after a DP. Two spreader grafts are placed and sutured at the dorsal part of the septum higher than the septum in its supratip location, usually obliquely to be lower on the septum more cephalically, without extending far in it's cephalic aspect. Those spreader grafts lift the

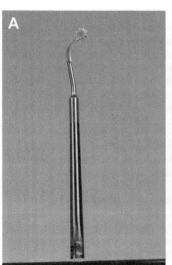
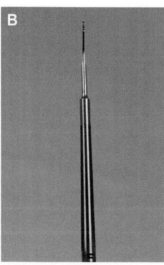

Fig. 11. (*A, B*) The long fan saw. This saw is used for closed lateral osteotomies, but it is also useful for cutting the bony septum, especially in portions where it is thick as frequently for the vomer.

supratip segment of the STP. Those spreader grafts can be extended caudally to add an end to end septal extension graft.

Lateralization of the Osseocartilaginous Vault (Lateral Push)

These are cases when a strong asymmetry of the bony pyramid makes its overall rotation desirable. In these cases, the osteotomies are that of a push down on one side (side where the nasal bones are the longest) and a let down on the other side. The precise ostectomy is easily performed at the naso-facial groove on the side where the bony vault must be rotated.

Bone wedge grafts placed in the lower part of lateral osteotomy make it possible to secure the final position of the bone pyramid.

Rhinosculpture is frequently used as an adjunc-tive procedure because the reliefs of the bony vault are generally different from the two sides and the rotation of the pyramid does not completely correct these differences in relief.

Realization of High Strips

Resections of bone septum are usually performed with mechanical instruments, especially with a gouge (or rongeur).[10] However, these instruments are used blindly and any twisting movement must be avoided so as not to destabilize the osteocarti-laginous junction of the septum.

The interest of piezo instruments for the resec-tion of the PPE is to make very precise cuts under direct visual control to avoid any radiated fracture at the skull base or toward the cartilaginous septum that could destabilize it. The preservation of septal stability is even more important when a significant septal harvesting will be made for the use of structural grafts. PEI allow to harvest signif-icant pieces of septum preserving the stability of the remaining L strut in high strip procedures.

Realization of Low Strips

Here too bone resections are usually made with a rongeur after disinsertion of the osteocartilaginous junction of the septum over its entire height. These resections concern the upper part of the PPE, the lower part of the vomer, and the anterior part of the bony septum.[11] However the bony septum trim-ming cane be done with piezo saws for a very pre-cise bone resection.

The use of piezo still allows one to perform all bone resections under direct visual control, and also avoids mucosal breaches. Bone incisions are made on the concave side of the bone.

The solid fixation of the septal flap to the anterior nasal spine is fundamental in this technique. The realization of a slit in the middle part of the anterior nasal spine with the right saw and holes on both sides thanks to the ultrasonic drill allows one to enclose the edge of the septum and to solidarize it in a solid way using nonresorbable sutures.

THE TECHNIQUE OF STRUCTURALLY RESHAPING THE DORSUM WITH PIEZOELECTRIC INSTRUMENTS

Hump removal according to traditional techniques has been the source of aesthetic and functional defects that have been greatly reduced by the reconstruction of the dorsum using spreader grafts and/or spreader flaps. However, even in these cases, small defects are not uncommon in the osseocartilaginous junction areas (dorsal and lateral keystone), an area where the often thin skin reveals all the defects either immediately or over time.

However, it is possible to avoid these defects thanks to a perfect bone resection in the keystone. This is done by rhinosculpture with ultrasonic rasps. Those inserts are essential to gradually remove the bony cap at the keystone areas, where this bone film is often thin, without damaging the ULC that will be used completely for the recon-struction of the dorsum. After the extended rhino-sculpture of the dorsal and lateral keystone areas, the ULC are incised tangentially to the septum, ris-ing much higher than if there had only been a tradi-tional rasping of the hump. This is when the roof is opened in a controlled way to be quickly closed in a controlled and solid way after septoplasty.

Lateral osteotomy is performed very low in the nasofacial groove from the Webster triangle to the highest part of the side wall, whenever it is necessary to reduce the base of the nose.

Paramedian osteotomy is performed whenever the width of the lateral keystone needs to be reduced. This osteotomy begins at the place where the ULC have been incised and oblique out-ward going toward the head of the eyebrow, to stop as high as possible on the nasal bone.

Finally, these two osteotomies are joined by a transverse osteotomy when the nasal pyramid re-mains too wide after the two previous osteoto-mies. This is usually the case when the bony vault is very broad or when the bones are stiff and strong.

A rhinosculpture adjunct is frequently needed to perfectly smooth the bone pyramid.

The new profile line is determined exactly by the resection of the septum to its dorsal part. Then the septoplasty is performed with the possibility to har-vest significant intact pieces of bone and cartilage if needed, and the middle third is reconstructed:

- At the most cephalic part, that is to say at the osseocartilaginous junction, the ULC are folded inside and positioned at the desired level with the help of needles. They are then sutured to the septum by use of PDS 5–0.
- Spreader grafts are positioned a little more caudal than usual, about 2 to 3 mm below the profile line, and they extend downward further than the anterior septal angle to make it possible to achieve an end-to-end septal extension graft.

The obliquity of spreader grafts is variable depending on whether one seeks to lower the entire profile line or lower the cephalic part but raise the caudal part.

The ULC are then sutured just above the spreader grafts, 1 mm under the edge of the septum (unless the middle third must be widened: the ULC are then sutured at the septum level). Needles are used to position ULC at the desired level and obliquity, and how these cartilages are sutured by the PDS points also determines the width of the middle third. The exact height of the profile line is therefore controlled, depending on what has been defined and the change in the position of the tip. Moreover the width of the STP is also determined by the way in which the ULC are sutured, but also by the cephalocaudal and lateral tension (depending on the folding of the ULC) that is put on these cartilages.

OTHER APPLICATIONS OF PIEZOELECTRIC INSTRUMENTS IN BONE CONTOURING OF THE NOSE
The Rhinosculpture of the Entire Bony Pyramid

Isolated rhinosculpture to correct a hump and a too wide bony pyramid is only possible when this pyramid is moderately too wide and the hump is modest (less than 2 mm). No osteotomy is then performed: the bony vault is generally reduced by the use of the scraper and rasps.

Removing the bony cap in the dorsal keystone area pops out the cartilaginous hump, which can actually become more pronounced than the original hump. The resection of the perichondrium at this level makes it possible to lower the profile line by 1 mm. If this is not enough, it is necessary to switch to a cartilaginous push down or if prefered to a foundation technique.

Crisscross Osteotomies

It is possible to correct excessive bone convexity by frame osteotomies. These crisscross osteotomies performed with a very thin saw make it possible to flatten a bone convexity while maintaining bone stability. They are rarely used, but their main indication is when there is convexity with very fine bones. If a rhinosculpture were used, it would result in a defect because of the thinness of the bones.

Some surgeons advocate the use of extended crisscross osteotomies on the sidewalls, but controlling the bone shape and stability may then be difficult.

ARE ELECTRICAL INSTRUMENTS COMPARABLE WITH PIEZOELECTRIC INSTRUMENTS?

Electrical instruments (eg, saws, rasps, burrs) share with PEI the advantage of not creating an unwanted fracture. However, these instruments are not selective: they cut or damage all tissues in contact with the insert. As a result, they can damage the supporting structures of the bones, but also cartilage, ligaments, and all subcutaneous tissues. Finally, the shape of the electric saws does not make it possible to adapt the path of the lateral osteotomies to the sinuosities of the nasaofacial groove. The endonasal approach of these lateral osteotomies means that the fracture line is located always higher (more dorsal) than the piezo lateral osteotomy performed in the nasofacial groove. This more lateral localization with the piezo allows for better bone stability.

The criticism often made to PEI of greater slowness does not hold for the nasal bones, which are generally thin and quickly remodeled or cut with piezo instruments, as soon as the adapted inserts are used.

DISCUSSION

Dorsum preservation techniques have developed to avoid the defects of classical hump reduction techniques (Joseph type) at the osseocartilaginous junction. To correct a hump, it is necessary to create an area of bone or osseocartilaginous weakness. This is either at the top of the pyramid, or a little lower at the bone cartilage junction, or at the base of the pyramid. The closer one gets to the top of the pyramid, the thinner the skin is in general and the more visible the defects can be.

The use of PEI in rhinoplasty has been a paradigm shift for bone remodeling. Thanks to the disruptive technology of piezo surgery, it has become possible to reshape the bones of the nose in a gentle and precise way, without creating a radiated fracture or bone instability. Initially, ultrasonic rhinoplasty allowed the correction of all types of humps and asymmetries of the nasal bones by stripping the bones on the hump area through extensive rhinosculpture, to transform the osseocartilaginous hump into a purely cartilaginous hump. It was then possible to simply reshape this hump by opening the septotriangular junction in a cephalic way, folding in the ULC and suturing them to the septum after redefining the dorsal profile line.

However, the versatility of this ultrasonic approach of the middle third that can be applied to all types of humps, all types of bones and cartilage has long been ignored, and the techniques of dorsal preservation have emerged to avoid the usual defects of the middle third, but also to facilitate the use of the closed rhinoplasty without having the difficulties related to the middle third reconstruction through a closed approach.

The structural hump reshaping with the PEI is based on bone and cartilaginous stability, to better control the fate of these structures. Structural techniques should preserve the bone stability with bone movements that are, depending on the location and direction of the osteotomies, rotation, translation, or lowering.

Conversely, the treatment of the hump and dorsum as part of dorsum preservation is based on bone instability, essential to bone impactions, that is, techniques acting on the base of the bone pyramid. For these techniques, the use of mechanical instruments that cause splinters and comminution at the fracture line is not a problem, because it facilitates bone lowering.

Foundation techniques in dorsum preservation (push down and let down) are based on bone sinking or lowering and require bone instability.

Preserving or restoring bone stability is not a purely theoretic, short- and long-term question:

- In the short term, bone instability can be the cause of an exaggerated bone collapse creating a step deformity, a residual hump, an asymmetry, or an axis defect of the bone pyramid.
- In the medium to long term, bone instability could create weakness, especially in case of shock, wearing heavy glasses, or certain masks.

PEI preserves bone stability by preserving the underlying bone support. We can imagine that the risk of deterioration, especially in the medium and long term, is reduced if bone stability is preserved or restored at the end of the operation.

PEI also makes it possible to perform all types of osteotomies on the bony pyramid and on the septum precisely without radiated fracture, regardless of the thickness and quality of the bone. This is notably useful for the PPE that must be precisely trimmed in high-strip and low-strip techniques.

Regarding the surface techniques of dorsum preservation (cartilaginous push down), the interest of the piezo is more to obtain a smooth osseocartilaginous transition at the keystone areas thanks to ultrasonic rasps. The use of fine ultrasonic saws also makes it possible to cut the bone precisely and imperceptibly on the dorsal or lateral keystone area, especially for techniques that preserve the bony cap in case of lowering of the hump.

SUMMARY

PEI allows novice or inexperienced surgeons to quickly master the different techniques of dorsum preservation or structural reshaping of the dorsum by avoiding several defects or complications. The realization of osteotomies, ostectomies, and rhinosculpture under direct visual control without risk of uncontrolled fracture allows a great precision and a great softness in the mobilization and the bone reshaping, for the preservation and structural management of the dorsum. PEI also helps to preserve bone stability and septum stability when cuts or bone remodeling are carried out appropriately.

Ultrasonic rhinoplasty and ultrasonic septoplasty have shown that they have a place for preservation rhinoplasty or structural rhinoplasty alongside more traditional techniques.

REFERENCES

1. Patel PN, Abdelwahab M, Most SP. A review and modification of dorsal preservation rhinoplasty techniques. Facial Plast Surg Aesth Med 2020;22(2): 71–9.
2. Gerbault O, Daniel RK, Palhazi P, et al. Reassessing surgical management of the bony vault in rhinoplasty. Aesth Surg J 2018;38:590–602.
3. Zholtikov V, Golovatinsky D, Palhazi P, et al. Rhinoplasty: a sequential approach to managing the bony vault. Aesth Surg J 2019;39:1–14.
4. Gerbault O, Daniel RK, Kosins AM. The role of piezoelectric instruments in rhinoplasty surgery. Aesth Surg J 2016;36:21–34.
5. Neves JC, Tagle DA, Dewes W, et al. A segmental approach in dorsal preservation rhinoplasty: the Tetris concept. Facial Plast Surg Clin North Am 2021; 29(1):85–99.

6. Kovacevic M, Veit JA, Toriumi D. Subdorsal Z flap; a modification of the Cottle technique in dorsal preservation rhinoplasty. Curr Opin Otolaryngol Head Neck Surg 2021;29(4). 544-251 2022,24(3).

7. IshidaLC, Ishida J, Ishida LH, et al. Nasal hump treatment with cartilaginous push down and preservation of the bony cap. Aesth Surg J 2020;40.

8. Ferreira MG, Monteiro D, Reis C, et al. Spare roof technique: a middle third new technique. Facial Plast Surg 2016;32(1):111–6.

9. Toriumi D. Subdorsal cantilever graft for elevating the dorsum in ethnic rhinoplasty. Facial Plast Surg Aesth Med 2022;24(3):143–59.

10. Saban Y, Daniel RK, Polselli R, et al. Dorsal preservation: the push down technique reassessed. Aesth Surg J 2018;38:117–31.

11. Cottle MH, Loring RM. Corrective surgery of the external nasal pyramid and the nasal septum for restauration of nasal physiology. Ill Med J 1946;90: 119–31.

Precision Segmental Preservation Rhinoplasty
Avoiding Widening, Defining New Dorsal Esthetic Lines in Dorsal Preservation Rhinoplasty

Jose Carlos Neves, MD[a],*, Ozan Erol, MD[b], Diego Arancibia-Tagle, MD[c], Emre Ilhan, MD[d]

KEYWORDS

- Preservation rhinoplasty • Segmental preservation • Precision rhinoplasty
- Dorsal platform preservation • DAL osteotomies • Tetris concept

 Video content accompanies this article at http://www.facialplastic.theclinics.com.

INTRODUCTION

Over the last decade, dorsal preservation rhinoplasty (PR) has regained an impressive popularity and has seen considerable advances in just a few years, as many doctors have improved and developed new ideas on the subject.[1]

In dorsal preservation, the initial fundament goal was to preserve both the keystone area (K-area) and the continuity of the cartilaginous vault. This conservative approach avoids nasal valve collapse, with its adverse effects on respiration and the dorsal esthetic lines (DALs).[2–4]

However, despite these "new" advances in the PR concept, we can still face some of the common drawbacks of this technique, such as hump recurrences, radix steps, supra-tip saddling, pyramid broadening, and lateralizations.[5,6]

Nasal pyramid widening or irregularities can be part of the drawbacks in dorsal PR. Some surgical options to correct a broad upper third (the bony pyramid) and irregularities in the upper/middle third have been described before.[6]

At the middle third (the cartilaginous vault), Stergiou and colleagues show that a widening can be advantageous as it opens the internal valve. They reported that internal nasal valve opening and nasal function can be dramatically improved by PR in a radiological analysis.[7] However, this condition may cause esthetic drawbacks. Saban and colleagues reported that excising a small strip from the caudal border of the upper lateral cartilages could solve the widening problem.[3]

The main concept to avoid drawbacks, as much as possible in dorsal preservation surgery, is to

Conflict of Interest Disclosures: None reported.

Funding Information: None of the authors have a financial interest in any of the products, devices, or drugs mentioned in this article.

Meeting Presentation: This research was presented at the 44th Annual Meetinf of European Academy of Facial Plastic Surgery Society; September 15-18, 2021; Nice, France.

[a] International and European Board Certified in Facial Plastic and Reconstructive Surgery (IBCFPRS - EBCFPRS), Private Practice at MYFACE Clinic and Academy, Lisbon, Portugal; [b] Head and Neck Surgery (FEBORL), Istanbul, Turkey; [c] International and European Board Certified in Facial Plastic and Reconstructive Surgery (IBCFPRS - EBCFPRS), Head and Neck Surgery (FEBORL). Private Practice, Mallorca, Spain; [d] International and European Board Certified in Facial Plastic and Reconstructive Surgery (IBCFPRS - EBCFPRS), Private Practice, Istanbul, Turkey

* Corresponding author.

E-mail address: jcneves@myface.pt

Facial Plast Surg Clin N Am 31 (2023) 155–170
https://doi.org/10.1016/j.fsc.2022.08.011

evaluate and treat the nose by segments and not as a single block, achieving a more predictable, accurate, and esthetically pleasing result.[6]

The segmental preservation approach encompasses five segments: the radix, the bony vault curvature, the rhinion, the pyramid vault curvature, and the supra-tip position, treating them as individual units to obtain a good result avoiding the most common problems in PR surgery.[6]

The use of power instruments such as Piezo and cylindrical burrs widely spread by Olivier Gerbault[8] and Emre Ilhan (Precision Rhinoplasty), respectively, is an important step in the segmental approach.

These burrs allow us to refine some irregularities in the osseocartilaginous framework, treat the lateral sidewalls bulging and asymmetries after the let-down maneuver, controlling the smoothness of the nasofacial groove, and precisely determine the DALs.

The concept of precision surgery has been described by other investigators,[9–11] but the main idea behind this precision segmental approach is to bring PR to another level of detail and finesse and to include in the PR some former contraindications.

This study also aims to show strategies we use to avoid the middle third widening and asymmetries in PR.

DORSAL PLATFORM PRESERVATION CONCEPT

Several classifications have been proposed for PR. Ferreira and colleagues[12] proposed a classification that would divide PR in foundation techniques and surface techniques. Although we believe conceptually identified with foundation techniques, in most cases we also end up performing procedures on the surface of the pyramid, such as sculpting with the use of burrs, piezo, or eventually rasps and adjustments of the cartilaginous pyramid (**Tables 1** and **2**). Therefore, we consider our work, our dorsal preservation (DP) *opera,* is divided into two acts: (1) the first act that is fundamentally the preparation of all the necessary conditions that make possible the impaction and reformulation of the nasal profile line when necessary (usually transforming convexity into flatness) and (2) the second act that is performed over the new position of the nasal pyramid and is dedicated to sculpt and to refine the bone and cartilage segments of the pyramid, in a precise way.

In some cases, in a smaller percentage, we end up not exposing the platform of the nasal dorsum during our dissection, keeping this area inviolate,

as we achieved the programmed profile only with the first act of deprojection and splaying of the dorsal profile line (**Fig. 1**A). However, in most cases, we need additional maneuvers to improve the nasal dorsum finesse, extending the dissection of the dorsal platform cephalically but avoiding the dissection of the radix as much as possible, a strategy that serves as an additional safety net to avoid a radix step phenomenon (**Fig 1**B). Exceptionally, we also dissect over the radix osteotomy line in cases we need to smooth the transition marked by the osteotomies or eventually to bring down the bone cephalic to the osteotomy for a better nasofrontal angle.

In our concept, our main goal is to maintain the continuity of the natural connection in between the nasal bone and the upper lateral cartilages (ULCs) on the dorsal platform, a platform that is defined laterally on both sides by the DALs, being our disarticulation work performed lateral to these lines. However, sculpture of the dorsal platform using preferably burrs can smooth the bone and cartilage, smoothing irregularities or solving convexities, in a considerable amount, without provoking disruption and therefore continuity impairment in between the bone of the upper third and the cartilage of the middle third, which would destroy the concept of preserving the anatomic continuity.

It was our observation during the years of consultation that, when talking about the nasal dorsum, the patients essentially value what they call the profile (which in reality is the $^3/_4$ view, because it is the view they evaluate when looking in the mirror) while palpating the dorsal platform. It is therefore essential to approach and define the DAL, which are evaluated in the $^3/_4$, and to achieve a smooth dorsal platform that on many occasions need precise sculpture and finesse, which allows the desired soft palpation. Our strategy will therefore aim to protect the base of the natural anatomy between these two esthetic lines and transfer the need for greater aggressiveness of the surgical gestures to the side walls lateral to the defined DAL, where healing problems are not usually experienced and where patients do not seem to encounter much displeasure.

PYRAMID REPOSITIONING AND BONE AND CARTILAGE BLOCKING POINTS

To understand the segmental concept when repositioning, the pyramid is paramount to clarify the blocking points of the bony and cartilaginous pyramid.

When performing impaction in foundation PR, two kinds of movements need to be considered

Table 1
Preservation rhinoplasty patients operated in the civil year 2021

	lateral wall approach			septal wall approach				dissection			sculpture with burr				reshaping bony DAL		reshaping cartilage DAL					supra-tip	radix
	let down	push down	LKA lls.articulation	tetris flap	lateral tetris	split tetris	low strip	lateral wall	dorsal platform	radix	lateral wall	dorsal bone	dorsal cartilage	radix	burr thinning	piezo osteotomy	ULC trimming	matress sutures	unilateral suture	spreader grafts	camouflage grafts	camouflage graft	camouflage graft
total	131	4	129	50	16	12	53	128	114	11	90	94	76	7	64	22	9	27	6	17	17	7	8
%	100,0%	03,5%	98,5%	38,2%	13,2%	9,1%	40,5%	97,7%	87,2%	8,4%	69,4%	71,6%	58,0%	5,3%	48,9%	16,8%	6,8%	20,6%	4,6%	12,9%	12,9%	5,3%	6,1%

Table 2
Precision segmental preservation rhinoplasty strategies

	Segmental Preservation	Precision Adjustment
Radix	• Avoiding radix area dissection when possible • Radix pillar • Step-up maneuver • Oblique radix osteotomy	• Osteotomy borders refinement (burr) • Deprojection the radix • Reduce radix with (burr)
Bony vault	• Avoiding dorsal platform dissection when possible • Let down avoiding blocking points • Radix pillar • Step-up maneuver	• Define the dorsal profile line (burr, piezo, rasps) • Define DAL width by re-shaping (burr) • New DAL osteotomies (piezo) • Lateral wall reshaping (burr) • Nasofacial groove reshaping (burr)

Rhinion	• Septal split (at the highest profile point)
	• LKA disarticulation
	• Sutures to counterbalance the spring effect
	  ◦ High strip with flap—Tetris flap to stable septum sutures
	  ◦ Low-strip approach—cable/mirror sutures in sub-laminar dissection
		• Reshaping bone cartilage transition (burr)

Cartilaginous vault	• Wide dissection posterior to the ULC
	• Scroll complex flap elevation to avoid the lower lateral cartilages (LLC) blocking point
	• Stabilizing the rotational movement with sutures
	  ◦ High strip with Tetris flap—flap to stable septum sutures
	  ◦ Low-strip approach—cable/mirror sutures in septal sub-laminar dissection
		• Cartilaginous vault running mattress sutures
		• Unilateral cartilaginous vault suture
		• Spreader and camouflage grafts
		• monopolar cautery reshaping new cartilaginous DALs and convexities

Supra-tip	• Supra-tip pillar ◦ High strip with Tetris flap—neural caudal septal strut bellow ULC • ULC caudal septal suture	• Supra-tip area burr shaving • Occasionally camouflage graft

(a) the vectorial deprojection movement—the anterior to posterior vectorial movement, when the pyramid is brought down to a new position but with preservation of the same profile contour, after preparing the three walls (two lateral walls and septum) to enable the impaction movement and (b) the rotational divergent movement during the bone/cartilage splaying, when a divergent movement of the bony and middle third lateral wall is created to flatten the dorsal contour, after creating the split maneuver in the three walls, with special attention to the lateral K-stone area disarticulation (**Fig. 2**)

During the impaction movement, the main *bony blocking points* are located at (1) the cephalic portion of the nasal septum (cephalic to the septal

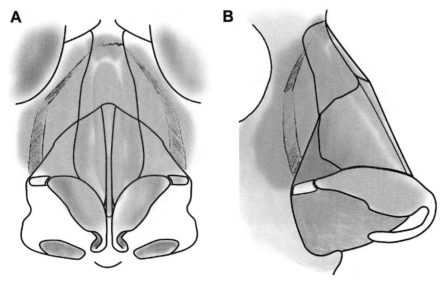

Fig. 1. (*A*) We always start dissecting the lateral wall reaching the nasofacial groove preserving the dorsal platform (blue); (*B*) when precision maneuvers are needed at the dorsal platform this region is dissected preserving the radix area (*purple gray*); exceptionally the radix area is exposed with the radix osteotomy being visible (*green*). The let-down osteotomies and the radix osteotomy can be seen.

split); (2) the lateral walls osteotomies contact, especially where the transverse and the lateral ones meet, allowing the posterior cephalic rotational movement of the bony pyramid; and (3) the inner lining mucosa must be seen as a possible bony blockage specially in push-down technique; the main *cartilaginous blocking points* are caused by (1) a deficient control of the septal cartilage caudal to the split, (2) the scroll complex, and (3) the soft tissues mass effect posterior to the ULC posterior border. The widening of the ULCs would not happen if their posterior and caudal borders were completely free. In that case they could move freely with the bony movement. So, it is important to understand the dissection posterior to the UCL posterior border and the role of the scroll by blocking the movement.

When dropping the pyramid down, most of the times, we create a divergence in between the bony wall and the mid-third wall. For that we

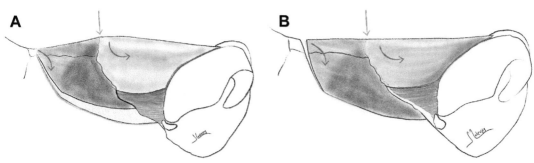

Fig. 2. Bone and cartilage lateral wall blocking points. Gray arrow represents the impaction vectorial force; the brown arrow represents the rotational forces of the pyramid: posterior and cephalic at the bony vault; caudal and anterior at the cartilaginous vault. The yellow line and shadow show where the bone will find the resistance; the green line and shadow represent the cartilaginous movement resistance. BONE: (*A*) the rotational movement happens around a radix stable pivotal point; if the pyramid finds blocking points (with special attention to the transverse osteotomy space and where it meets the basal osteotomies) a nondesired displacement of the radix osteotomy may occur (*B*); CARTILAGE: (*A*) the rotational movement is posterior and caudal toward the soft tissues posterior to the ULC posterior border and toward the scroll area, respectively. If these structures limit the ULC movement, they will find resistance (green *line* and shadow) and consequent bulging and widening will be seen (*B*). Lateral K stone area (LKA) disarticulation: the bone is released in a wide extension from the ULC, mucosa and pyriform ligament (this one the most limiting structure for the splaying effect (purple shadow).

Neves et al

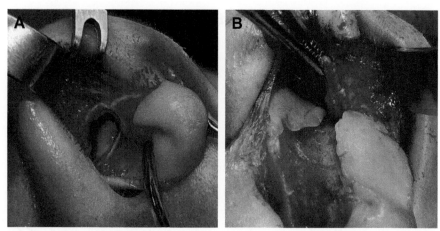

Fig. 3. Elevating the scroll complex with the soft tissues flap. (*A*) The sesamoid cartilages can be seen in the flap; (*B*) when both horizontal and vertical scroll ligaments are elevated the mucosa is the only lawyer left behind. It creates space for the ULC rotational movement.

need to disarticulate the bony nasal wall from the ULC and release the pyriform ligament from the pyriform aperture[13] (**Fig. 3**). This maneuver allows the caudal and anterior advancement of the middle third promoting some stretching, which works as additional measure for narrowing but it does not work as a blocking point, once the free bony movement brings the cartilage down precisely with the same width, if the other cartilaginous were released.

Materials and Methods

We analyzed retrospectively our 2021 rhinoplasty data. We performed 321 operations, of which 208 were primary and 113 were revision rhinoplasties. The revision ones were excluded. Of the 208 primary rhinoplasties, the ones based in structure concepts (77) were also excluded, remaining the 131 cases operated with PR concepts. We first analyzed the work of the lateral and medial walls that promote the reposition of the pyramid and the remodeling of the dorsal profile based on the segmental PR concept. This is the "act 1" of our PR approach. In some cases, only the lateral wall is dissected avoiding the manipulation of the dorsal platform soft tissues, which can benefit the post-op recovery for inducing less traumas. However, in most cases, we end up dissecting the dorsal platform to perform refinement maneuvers to the profile and precisely define the DAL. These maneuvers at the bony and pyramid vaults that represent the "act 2" were also recorded, to understand the importance of modifying the original characteristics of the nasal pyramid, which allow to include in our PR surgical list former classical contraindication cases.

SURGICAL TECHNIQUE

In our routine, we start approaching the lateral wall, in a subareolar (supra-perichondral) plane in the lower and middle thirds and subperiosteal in the upper third in a wide approach manner,[14] so the nasal facial groove is reached but with no dorsal platform soft tissues elevation. This extended dissection allows us to perform the lateral wall procedures under direct vision and a free movement of all tissues avoiding the mass effect of the soft tissues blockage to the ULCs. The dorsal platform is addressed and dissected if some additional refinement maneuvers are considered in that area, which we frequently do.

We need to properly address why the middle vault widens during PR. If the middle third cartilages were free in space with no contact to other structures, they would not change the form and width when any kind of movement was applied. It means that the potential blocking points are some ULC neighbors. We believe that the scroll areas and all soft tissues posterior to the ULC are important blocking points in the impaction maneuver. (LKAs and pyriform ligaments are limitation structures for the rotational splaying effect but do not cause widening if not released.) Therefore, one must separate these structures; otherwise, they limit the movement holding the middle vault to exhibit a convexity on the outer surface of the upper lateral cartilages, leading to a widening effect, as well as hump recurrences.

In addition, as the cartilaginous vault experiences a caudal and anterior rotational movement, the scroll areas and the supra-tip region may be compressed with a consequent conflict and a possible bulging. To avoid this effect, we elevate and preserve the scroll complex during our

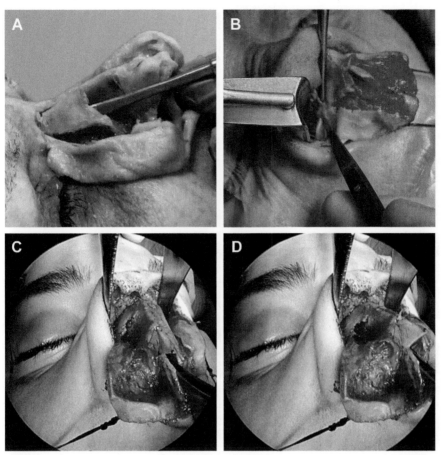

Fig. 4. LKA disarticulation. (*A*) Wide dissection in a cadaveric specimen; (*B*) the resistance of the pyriform ligament, the most limiting element for the splaying movement. We use a scissors to cut it from the pyriform apertura. Note the disarticulation area before the rotational movement (*C*) and the opening of the joint after right after (*D*) It shows the importance of having this connection released.

dissection, and eventually, a caudal trimming of the ULCs at the end of the surgery is necessary.

ACT 1: Releasing and repositioning the nasal pyramid and formatting the dorsal profile line

Scroll Area Dissection

In the closed or open approaches, we start by dissecting the inner surface of both medial crura in a supra-perichondral plane without damaging the soft tissues in between. We proceed toward the domes and reaching the lateral crura. At this stage, we dissect the outer surface of the lateral crura keeping the supra-perichondral subareolar plane with a delicate elevator reaching the cephalic margin of the cartilage. The scroll complex is identified and elevated with the soft tissues flap. The scroll region mucosa is consequently exposed (see **Fig. 3**). Preservation of the scroll complex can be achieved by a sub-perichondral or a subareolar dissection. We believe that the elevation of the scroll ligament complex control is the first step to avoid ULC widening.

Regardless of the dissection philosophy used, the ULC movement should not encounter resistance.

Wide Lateral Wall Dissection

As already described, the wide dissection allows the pyramid to move posteriorly without the compression of the lateral wall tissues, making the lateral wall wide dissection (eventually keeping the dorsal platform soft tissues intact no elevated) important not only for exposure and visibility of the framework structures but also for the free pyramid repositioning movement. We usually dissect laterally to the nasal facial groove. By exposing this area, we can manage not only the shape of the bony lateral wall but also the angle and the softness of the groove with great precision.

Lateral Keystone Area Disarticulation and Pyriform Ligament Release

Before starting the LKA disarticulation, we perform the lateral let-down (occasionally push-down)

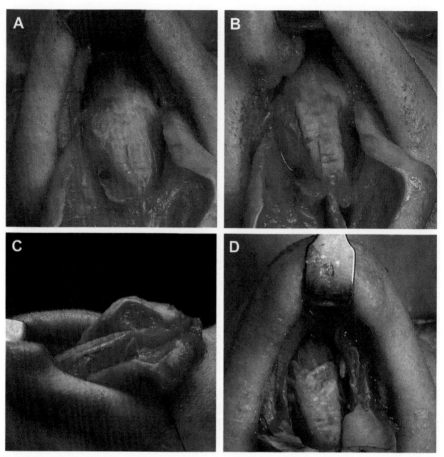

Fig. 5. (*A*) Broad nasal dorsum; (*B*) and (*C*) continuous mattress sutures with reduction of the ULC flaring; (*D*) new DAL were designed narrowing the bony vault with a cylindrical burr. Note the continuity of bony and cartilaginous esthetic lines. Compare the width in (*A*) and (*D*), before and after.

osteotomies and remove the bone wedges by protecting both outer and inner periosteum. LKA disarticulation (lateral split maneuver[15] or Ballerina maneuver[16]) refers to elevate the lateral bony wall from the ULC, elevating the inner periosteum of the lateral wall with a Freer, and even more important sectioning the pyriform ligament from all its attachments to the bony pyriform aperture (the most limiting structure for flattening the dorsal profile), with a scissors, always avoiding mucosal damage (**Fig. 4**). At this stage, it is essential to avoid dorsal K-area dissection not to disturb the stabilization.

Now, we are able to move the nasal pyramid to the desired position and flattening the dorsum as predicted.

*ACT 2:*Maneuvers to prevent residual humps and irregularities and to prevent widening and promote narrowing and definition.

Suturing the Middle Third Roof

The middle third roof suturing goal is to narrow a wide middle third roof and get a precision dorsal

line by preserving nasal functions in rhinoplasty. After the nasal dorsum projection is reduced and stabilization is achieved, the dorsal line harmony should be checked. If there is broadening or asymmetry on the middle third roof despite all the maneuvers, the suturing option should be considered.

Continuous or intermittent 5.0 polydiaxonone suture (PDS) sutures can be used starting a few millimeters cephalically from the W-point running cephalically. When a continuous horizontal mattress suture is performed, we turn caudally again and tie the suture at the starting point (**Fig. 5**).

For the patients who have broader cartilages, we need to excise a triangular piece of cartilage at the dorsal T platform starting at the rhinion (the base of the triangle), in between the septum and the thickest aspect of the ULC, going caudally till necessary (the apex of the triangle). The three components, the two ULC and septum, are brought together achieving the ideal width. The suture described above can be applied now if necessary. In other

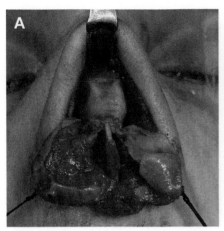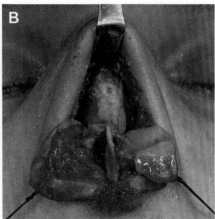

Fig. 6. (*A*) Wide and irregular middle third; (*B*) continuous mattress sutures; note the trimming of the ULC edges next to the rhinion area: also new DAL were created with piezo (note the green-stick osteotomy in both sides) and shaved with a cylindrical burr.

cases, trimming the edge of the ULC close to the rhinion may prevent cartilage irregularities (**Fig. 6**). The use of monopolar cautery can also be an interesting option to control these edges. Moreover, its use can reduce some convexity of the ULC lateral wall and still allow to sculpt new cartilaginous DALs.

There are a few critical points to help avoiding drawbacks of the technique. The suture should be placed as more anterior as possible, close to the T platform (see **Fig. 5**C), where the ULC are thicker to avoid collapse of the middle third lateral wall and eventual consequent breathing problems, what can happen if the suture is performed in a more posterior position.

Also, the suture should save a free segment next to the nasal bones to avoid excessive narrowing of the middle third next to the rhinion, which can lead to an apparent pyriform aperture and a consequent inverted V aspect. In addition, the suture should be tightened according to the desired dorsal lines. Too tight or too loose may produce non-ideal esthetic lines. Based on that, in some cases is preferable to use single sutures.

In some cases, only one ULC is bulging, specifically if we are dealing with a crooked nose. A single unilateral suture can be placed using the same concept. The knot can be buried in the depression found in between the septum and upper lateral; it is interestingly well disguised in this area.

Precision Pyramid Sculpting

The precision structure rhinoplasty concepts referring to the use of power instruments to refine the nasal pyramid may play a relevant role to deliver

precise a designed dorsum, esthetic dorsal lines, and smooth lateral walls in PR.

Both ultrasonic devices (the piezo) and burrs may be used to shave the dorsum. Even rasps can smooth some bony dorsum details. We use mainly diamond cylindrical burrs to correct irregular areas while removing the hump and reducing the lateral walls. As demonstrated by Emre Ilhan, the cylindrical burr because of its larger contact area compared with the spherical burr creates a smoother bony surface with less probability to produce grooves or irregularities. Even regarding the piezo scraper, the cylindrical burr shows this advantage.

Reshaping dorsal residual humps

It is common to see after the impaction and splaying maneuvers a residual bony hump, mainly in an S-shape bony dorsum.[17] There has been this discussion regarding indications and algorithms to address kyphotic noses and S-shape bony vaults seen as relative contraindications for foundation techniques. In fact, in most of our cases after our foundation maneuver, we do surface procedures with the burrs being a main character. The residual bony hump created by the S-shape bone is sculpt till the desired level. In some cases, even the cartilaginous vault has some irregularities and some convexity. Even if we need to have in mind not to disrupt the dorsal K-area, this connection is of great stability and we have been pushed it to the limit without ever seen any disruption. This maneuver allows till 2 mm at both bony pyramid and cartilaginous pyramid reduction, which allows a great control and precision of the profile line after the impaction technique. The burr has again a great advantage over the piezo when addressing the

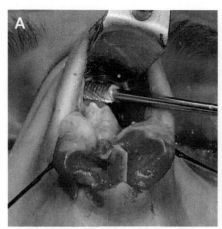
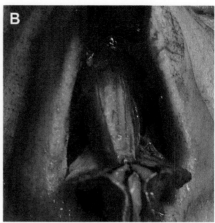

Fig. 7. (*A*) The cylindrical burrs flatten and smooth the dorsal platform; (*B*) the ULC perichondrium was partially drilled showing the ULC cartilaginous shoulders; this maneuver can deproject the cartilaginous dorsum till 2 mm.

cartilage. Piezo does not have the ability to modify cartilage, whereas the cylindrical burr can effectively shave perichondrium and cartilage (**Fig. 7**)

Sculpting the lateral wall

The lateral wall can be also sculpted. It is common to see some bulging of the lateral wall at the nasofacial groove. This bulging may be completely or partially corrected by the let-down wedge resection, when some building remains the burr can be used to smooth its convexity. In deviated noses, PR can be real powerful bringing the pyramid to the midline. However, in many cases, the lateral walls remain asymmetric, with convexities or concavities, which can be corrected with the use of power instruments.[18,19] Both walls can be shaved till the inner cortical of the lateral is observed as a gray granite look. This paper-thin bone can be remodeled by digital compression, a powerful tool to control bony convexities (**Fig. 8**).

The nasofacial groove is also addressed. In many occasions, after the basal osteotomies, some steps can be felt at this point. The use of the burr smooths the basal edge of the osteotomy, creating a gentle transition to the face and helping in reducing the width of the nasal base (**Fig. 9**).

The width is defined, and a new DAL is designed. Its continuity with the cartilaginous vault may be also shaved. In some cases, the shaving limit is reached, leaving only an eggshell thickness of lateral bone but still with some undesired dorsal width. In these cases, we may consider DAL osteotomies.

Defining dorsal esthetic lines osteotomies

In wider bony vaults, the reshape of the DALs can also be achieved with power instruments,[20] performing DAL osteotomies that should be placed immediately lateral to where we would like to see the new DAL, so the dorsal platform has the adequate width and continues smoothly with the cartilaginous vault. This is the main goal of our approach in dorsal PR to preserve the dorsum in between the (new) DAL leaving the main trauma (that necessarily exists) to the lateral wall where really few complications must be seen and almost never irregularities are palpated. These DAL osteotomies should not traverse the entire thickness of the bone, but rather create a groove along the fracture line allowing for a greenstick fracture that aids in the stability of the lateral bone wall. Because after the let-down maneuverer the nasal pyramid has some instability, here the use of piezo is for sure of a high value by creating a precise cut. Sometimes by fragilizing this area with the burr, the bone becomes paper thin as already mentioned and the lateral wall fractures in at the defined DAL (see **Fig. 8** and **Fig. 10**). Thus, we defined precisely the width of the dorsal platform, control the surface of the lateral wall and fracture it in to narrow the bony nasal base. With these technical possibilities, the contraindication for PR is at least only a partial contraindication if any.

Grafting the Middle Third

It is commonly seen, especially in deviated pyramids, that the middle third may show asymmetric ULC with eventual concavity of their outer surface. Like in structure rhinoplasty, some grafts can be placed to help solving these problems. In crooked noses, the ULC contralateral to the deviation is often observed concave. On many occasions, when the pyramid is centered in the midline and the septum is straight, this concavity solves naturally. In other occasions, the concavity remains

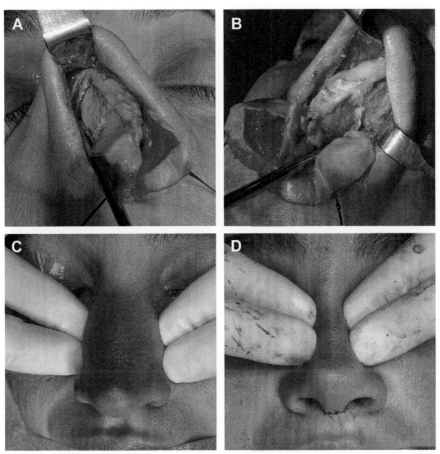

Fig. 8. (*A*) and (*B*) In this case, the lateral bony wall was shaved till a gray granite look is observed; the bone is paper-thin in some regions. The width of the dorsal platform was reduced to the ideal measurement creating a new DAL; the piezo helped creating a green-stick fracture; a continuous mattress sutures was place at the cartilaginous vault; (*C*) pre-op dorsal width; (*D*) immediate post-op width.

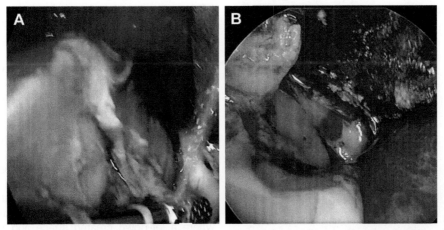

Fig. 9. (*A*) Left lateral nasal wall, where it is visible the gap left by the let-down technique. The edge of the basal osteotomy border is sharp. Even if the osteotomy in very low at the nasofacial groove it can eventually be palpated; (*B*) after smoothing the transition with the cylindrical burr.

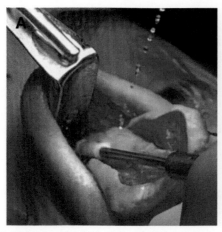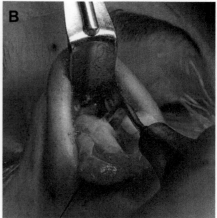

Fig. 10. (*A*) Reshaping the DAL with a drill; (*B*) defining the new DAL with a piezo.

with the need of correction to adjust the esthetic line and the lateral wall depression. For this, we have two options:

Use of spreader graft

A submucosal pocket can be defined to place the spreader graft in place to pop out the concave ULC; other option is to separate caudally the ULC from the septum and insert a spreader to define precisely the mid-wall DAL (**Fig. 11**).

Use of camouflage graft

In some cases, it is easier to use a camouflage graft that is made of cartilage, perichondrium, fascia, or other option. The graft should recreate the continuity of the DAL and/or give volume to the concave ULC. When this approach is chosen, attention to functional details of the mid-third is important.

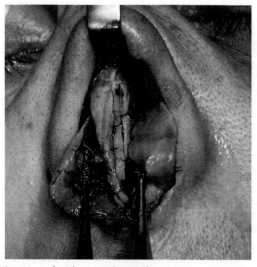

Fig. 11. Left side spreader graft.

DISCUSSION

In 2018, the first author had the opportunity of sharing some surgical techniques concepts in a cadaveric laboratory with the coauthor Emre Ilhan. Precision rhinoplasty referring to the use of burrs in structure rhinoplasty produced a brainstorming that would definitely import new tools to PR that would change indications and quality of the results. Dorsal platform preservation and DAL design are a strategy that aims to achieve the best natural result without the need for reconstruction, avoiding eventual numerous problems that rebuilding the sectioned dorsum may eventually show during the long run.

However, as with dorsal structure surgery, preservation of the nasal dorsum can result in stigmata, characteristic of the technique, when not properly performed or without due care in detail, as already stated.

As any other surgical procedure or technique, PR has its own relative and absolute contraindications. It is also surgeon-dependent, what makes the approach variability truly wide. As an example, Yves Saban published his personal very well elaborated algorithm[21] that does not overlap in many concepts our logic of approach. This range of options, personal indications, and variability of noses make this article of rhinoplasty really challenging.

In our series of PR in 2021 (see **Table 1**), we performed let-down technique in all patients and except four patients (3.5%) that presented marked deviated pyramids, and we performed a push-down maneuver in the ipsilateral wall of the deviation to tilt the pyramid to the contralateral side where a let-down created space and facilitates the movement, all the other patients had a bilateral let-down.

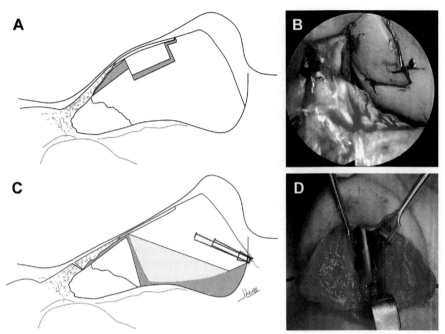

Fig. 12. (*A*) and (*B*) High-strip with Tetris cartilaginous flap; (*C*) and (*D*) low-strip with cable sutures (mirror sutures).

Only in two patients that presented a high straight dorsum we did not disarticulate the LKA. In 98.5% of the cases, it was performed to promote effectively the splaying effect in between the upper third and middle third lateral walls.

As mentioned, we base our work in foundation techniques being the high strip with a cartilaginous flap (the Tetris block) (**Fig. 12**A, Video 1) and the low strip our choices when adopting PR. We performed 78 Tetris flaps (59.5%) with its variations, our favorite choice whenever possible because

of the stabilization and definition of the position of the pyramidal segments over a stable basal septum, and 53 low-strip approaches (40.5%) (**Fig. 12**C) always a choice in more severe pyramid or septal deviations where the Tetris flap technique may limit the capacity of correction. To increase the stability of our free low-strip flap, we perform a sub-laminar (supra-perichondral) (**Fig. 13**) nasal septum dissection to increase the resistance to the cheese-wired effect produced by the sutures settled to the anterior nasal spine

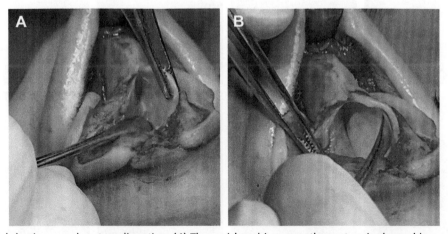

Fig. 13. Sub-laminar nasal septum dissection. (*A*) The perichondrium over the septum is observable as well as the dissection plane elevation the lamina propria; (*B*) the bloodless fields shows clearly the perichondrium and the lamina propria.

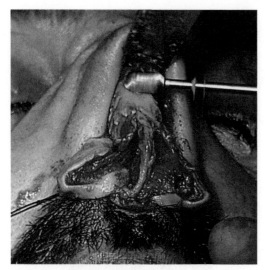

Fig. 14. Refining the cartilaginous surface with a cylindrical burr.

(ANS). The increase of resistance is dramatic (Video 2). To add another level of pyramid position accuracy, we block the septal wall using cable sutures that are placed in both sides of the ANS (mirror sutures when symmetric) that stabilize in a 3D perspective and oblique cables oriented from the ANS to the rhinion that following the counterbalance force concept developed in the subdorsal Tetris will stabilize effectively the rhinion position (see **Fig. 12**C, D).

We start our dissection of the lateral nasal wall after elevating the scroll complex sparing at this moment the midline dorsal platform. However, because what really matters is the finesse of the result in 87.2% of the patients we decided to perform other additional direct maneuvers and elevated the dorsal soft tissues as well. Yet, avoidance of the radix was the rule. Only in 11 cases (8.4%) it was exposed, to sculpt it with burrs in seven cases and to place a radix graft in eight cases, two of which were to correct an iatrogenic step-down deformity.

The use of power instruments and specifically the use of burrs have changed considerably the indications for PR. In our casuistic, we used the burr to flatten a still convex bony vault in 94 cases (71.6%). It shows that if this area is not addressed in a high percentage of patients, we will contraindicate foundation PR in some cases (like kyphotic noses) or will end up with residual bony humps or irregularities. The cartilaginous pyramid was also shaved to a more refined profile line in more than half of the patients (76 patients, 58%) what shows how this segment can be more convex than we eventually value and proves the effectiveness of the burr working in cartilage (see **Fig. 7**B; **Fig. 14**).

Based on the review of the literature, a wide nasal pyramid is one of the most important contraindications for dorsal preservation surgery. Moreover, it was previously emphasized that this

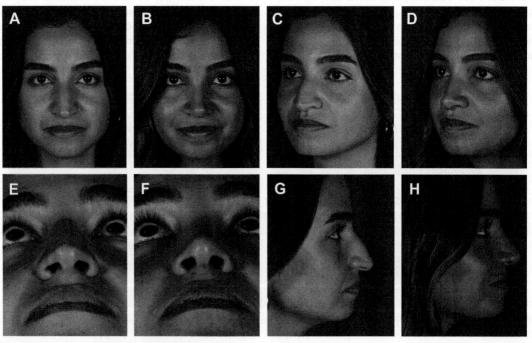

Fig. 15. Pre op (*A,C,E,F*), Post op (*B,D,F,H*).

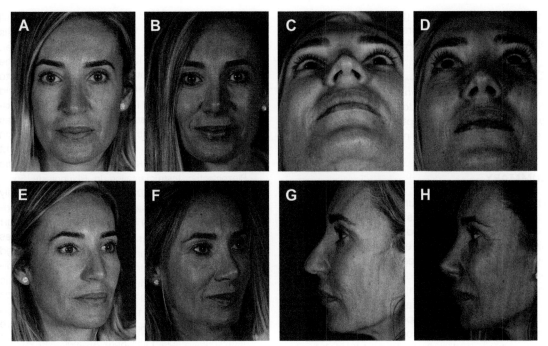

Fig. 16. Pre op (*A,C,E,F*), Post op (*B,D,F,H*).

technique could be performed in patients with a wish to widen the vault. However, we show strategies that can avoid widening of the middle vault and even more can make them narrower without disruption of its stability. Understanding the cartilaginous blocking points is paramount. Free the posterior and caudal borders of the ULCs and disarticulate it from the bone at the LKA allows the middle vault to rotate anterior and caudal and assume its new position without distortion. Nevertheless, in some cases, we started from an already wide or irregular dorsum that depends mostly in the ULCs flare. In those cases, dorsal cartilaginous platform sutures can correct this deformity. Bilateral mattress sutures (27 patients) and unilateral sutures (6 patients) were used effectively in one-quarter of the patients. More rarely some cartilage trimming was done specifically around the rhinion area, as we prefer to use the burrs in cartilage irregularities. Other option is to use a monopolar cautery burning the prominent cartilage which leaves no depression or irregularity. In asymmetric pyramids, in a clear association with the low-strip approach, a control of the cartilaginous DAL was achieved by using a unilateral spreader graft or a camouflage graft (17 patients both).

Probably the most exciting tool that we add to the bony dorsum control is the definition of new DAL following the principle that we preserve the nasal dorsal platform and transfer the work to the nasal lateral wall. Therefore, we frequently work

on the lateral wall with burrs to define the surface and to smooth the nasofacial groove (90% of the cases). These two surfaces, lateral wall and bony vault, are now starting to define the DAL. This DAL can be shifted to a more central position (narrowing the dorsum) by thinning the bone with burrs that may eventually provoke a paper-thin bone that fractures-in (we performed it half of our patients) or by designing it using a piezo, which also creates a green-stick in-fracture (16.8%). These power instruments can design with great precision the width of the dorsum, the drawing of the DAL, the position of the lateral wall, and the smoothness of the nasofacial groove.

It is another perspective of foundation PR that allows us to control the width of the nasal pyramid, preserving the dorsal platform and designing precisely where the DAL ideally will be seen, conditions that focus our patients' concerns, observing a precise $^3/_4$ view and palpating a smooth dorsum with no transition areas or surface interruptions. Strategically, a great amount of the surface work is transferred to the lateral wall where it is very difficult to point relevant problems.

CLINICAL CASES
Case Study 1

Dorsal PR work: let-down technique and LKA disarticulation; right side overlap lateral Tetris flap; lateral wall sculpted with 5 mm cylindrical burr; DAL refined by piezo, green-stick osteotomy; continuous mattress suture at the cartilaginous platform, 5.0 PDS (**Fig. 15**A–H).

Case Study 2

Dorsal PR work: let-down technique and LKA disarticulation; septal subdorsal Tetris flap; lateral wall and bony dorsum sculpted with 5 mm cylindrical burr; cartilaginous continuous mattress suture, 5.0 PDS (**Fig. 16**A–H).

SUMMARY

The dorsal preservation surgery, which has been popular in recent years, is increasing its magic. Despite its reputation, the drawbacks of this technique should not be ignored. To avoid the nasal pyramid widening and irregularities and achieve precise DAL in PR, we need to consider additional maneuvers apart from impacting and splaying. Following this principle in a considerable number of our patients, we end up performing surface procedures, additional osteotomies as DAL osteotomies, sutures, and grafts to the mid-third. It leads to the question: what are we really preserving? The answer guided the logic of this article: the nasal dorsal platform continuity with precisely defined DAL.

SUPPLEMENTARY DATA

Supplementary data related to this article can be found online at https://doi.org/10.1016/j.fsc.2022.08.011.

REFERENCES

1. Neves JC, Tagle DA, Dewes W, et al. A Segmental Approach in Dorsal Preservation Rhinoplasty: The Tetris Concept. Facial Plast Surg Clin North Am 2021;29(1):85–99.
2. Arancibia-Tagle D, Neves JC, D'Souza A. History of Dorsum Conservative Techniques in Rhinoplasty: The Evolution of a Revived Technique. Facial Plast Surg 2021;37(1):86–91.
3. Saban Y, Daniel RK, Polselli R, et al. Dorsal preservation: the push down technique reassessed. Aesthet Surg J 2018;38(02):117–31.
4. Saban Y, Braccini F, Polselli R. Morphodynamic anatomy of the nose. In: Saban Y, Braccini F, Polselli R, et al, editors. Paris: The Monographs of CCA Group; 2002. p. 25–32, 32.
5. Ferraz MBJ, Sella GCP. Indications for Preservation Rhinoplasty: Avoiding Complications. Facial Plast Surg 2021;37(1):45–52.
6. Neves JC, Arancibia-Tagle D. Avoiding Aesthetic Drawbacks and Stigmata in Dorsal Line Preservation Rhinoplasty. Facial Plast Surg 2021;37(1):65–75.
7. Stergiou G, Tremp M, Finocchi V, et al. Functional and Radiological Assessment After Preservation Rhinoplasty - A Clinical Study. Vivo 2020;34(5):2659–65.
8. Gerbault O, Daniel RK, Kosins AM. The Role of Piezoelectric Instrumentation in Rhinoplasty Surgery. Aesthet Surg J 2016;36(1):21–34.
9. Macdonald JA. Precision rhinoplasty. Plast Reconstr Surg 1988;82(4):728–9.
10. Guyuron B. Precision rhinoplasty. Part I: The role of life-size photographs and soft-tissue cephalometric analysis. Plast Reconstr Surg 1988;81(4):489–99.
11. Guyuron B. Precision rhinoplasty. Part II: Prediction. Plast Reconstr Surg 1988;81(4):500–5.
12. Gonçalves Ferreira M, Toriumi DM. A Practical Classification System for Dorsal Preservation Rhinoplasty Techniques. Facial Plast Surg Aesthet Med 2021;23(3):153–5.
13. Rohrich RJ, Hoxworth RE, Thornton JF, et al. The pyriform ligament. Plast Reconstr Surg 2008;121(1):277–81.
14. Zholtikov V, Golovatinsky V, Palhazi P, et al. Rhinoplasty: A Sequential Approach to Managing the Bony Vault. Aesthet Surg J 2020;40(5):479–92.
15. Neves JC, Arancibia Tagle D, Dewes W, et al. The split preservation rhinoplasty: "the Vitruvian Man split maneuver". Eur J Plast Surg 2020;43:323–33.
16. Goksel A, Saban Y, Tran KN. Biomechanical Nasal Anatomy Applied to Open Preservation Rhinoplasty. Facial Plast Surg 2021;37(1):12–21.
17. Lazovic GD, Daniel RK, Janosevic LB, et al. Rhinoplasty: the nasal bones - anatomy and analysis. Aesthet Surg J 2015;35(3):255–63.
18. Becker DG, Toriumi DM, Gross CW, et al. Powered instrumentation for dorsal reduction. Facial Plast Surg 1997;13(4):291–7.
19. Davis RE, Raval J. Powered instrumentation for nasal bone reduction: advantages and indications. Arch Facial Plast Surg 2003;5(5):384–91.
20. Davis RE, Foulad AI. Treating the Deviated or Wide Nasal Dorsum. Facial Plast Surg 2017;33(2):139–56.
21. Saban Y, de Salvador S. Guidelines for Dorsum Preservation in Primary Rhinoplasty. Facial Plast Surg 2021;37(1):53–64.

Moving?

Make sure your subscription moves with you!

To notify us of your new address, find your **Clinics Account Number** (located on your mailing label above your name), and contact customer service at:

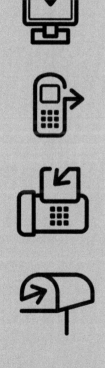

Email: journalscustomerservice-usa@elsevier.com

800-654-2452 (subscribers in the U.S. & Canada)
314-447-8871 (subscribers outside of the U.S. & Canada)

Fax number: 314-447-8029

**Elsevier Health Sciences Division
Subscription Customer Service
3251 Riverport Lane
Maryland Heights, MO 63043**

ELSEVIER

Printed and bound by CPI Group (UK) Ltd, Croydon, CR0 4YY

08/05/2025

01864717-0012